# Studying Those
# Who Study Us

# WRITING SCIENCE

EDITORS  Timothy Lenoir and Hans Ulrich Gumbrecht

# Studying Those Who Study Us

AN ANTHROPOLOGIST
IN THE WORLD OF
ARTIFICIAL INTELLIGENCE

*Diana E. Forsythe*

EDITED, WITH AN INTRODUCTION, BY *David J. Hess*

STANFORD UNIVERSITY PRESS
STANFORD, CALIFORNIA
2001

Stanford University Press
Stanford, California

© 2001 by the Board of Trustees of the
Leland Stanford Junior University

Printed in the United States of America
on acid-free, archival-quality paper

Library of Congress Cataloging-in-Publication Data

Forsythe, Diana
    Studying those who study us : an anthropologist in the
world of artificial intelligence / Diana E. Forsythe ;
edited, with an introduction, by David J. Hess.
        p.    cm. — (Writing Science)
    Includes bibliographical references and index.
    ISBN 0-8047-4141-7 (alk. paper) —
    ISBN 0-8047-4203-0 (pbk. : alk. paper)
    1. Ethnology—Methodology.    2. Artificial intelligence—
Social aspects.    3. Information technology—Social aspects.
4. Medical informatics.    5. Medical anthropology.
6. Feminist anthropology.    I. Hess, David J.    II. Title.
III. Series.
GN34.3.I53 F67    2001
306'.01—dc21                                     2001020018

Original Printing 2001

Last figure below indicates year of this printing:
10    09    08    07    06    05    04    03    02    01

Designed by Janet Wood
Typeset by James P. Brommer in 10/14 Sabon
and Helvetica Black display

# CONTENTS

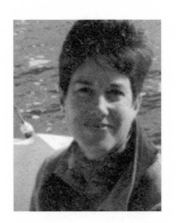

In August 1997 Diana Forsythe drowned while crossing a fifty-foot-wide river on a vacation in Alaska. The tour guide of the hiking group, who was an old friend, apparently realized that the river had become swollen to dangerous levels, and he motioned some of the hikers in the party to turn back. Diana lost her footing, slipped out of her backpack, and struggled to swim to a sand bar, but she was carried away by the current. Fellow hikers in the tour found her body about a mile down the river.

The shock of Diana's death reverberated through the communities of people who knew her. She had studied or worked in several universities in North America and Europe, and she was known in many professional circles, including feminist science studies; the anthropology of science, technology, and work; European studies; and medical informatics. At the 1997 annual meeting of the American Anthropological Association, several of her colleagues expressed both their personal grief and their sense of intellectual loss for a founder and leader in the anthropology of science, technology, and work. Colleagues were concerned that some of Diana's research, especially the unpublished papers, might become lost. This book is a collective effort that emerged out of the general sense among her colleagues that it was important to rescue her last writings in the anthropology of science, technology, and work and to make them generally available.

Diana played an important intellectual role as a founder of the subfield of the anthropology of science and technology, and she also helped articulate the field with the anthropology of work and with feminist science studies. The prize that now bears her name is suggestive of the contribution she made: "The prize celebrates the best book or series of published articles in the spirit of Diana Forsythe's feminist anthropological research on work, science, and/or technology, including biomedicine." Diana's feminism was muted in her first publications in the anthropology of science and technology, as will be evident in the opening chapters of this volume, but it was becoming increasingly evident in the papers she was working on before her untimely death. Indeed, the chapters in this book reveal the gradual unfolding of an active mind and growing research program. As readers progress through the chapters and witness the development of her thinking, they will begin to appreciate the intellectual loss felt by her community of peers.

The papers collected in this volume focus on her contribution to the anthropology of science and technology, but it is important to remember that she also contributed to two other areas of research: European studies and medical informatics. In the area of European studies, she did fieldwork in Scotland, where she contributed to the literatures on migration and education, and in Germany, where she studied national identity. Her research on the latter topic became one of the starting points for a conference called "Inspecting Germany," held in Tübingen in 1998. Some of Diana's work on medical informatics is included here, but she also wrote or coauthored several more technical articles that were published in medical informatics and expert systems publications. As will be evident from the later chapters in the book, she was having an impact on the knowledge acquisition methods used in the field. Although the European studies and the medical informatics papers written for technical journals are not gathered in this volume, they are listed in the appendix and bibliography.

DIANA'S LIFE

The Internet domain name of <@forsythe.stanford.edu> attests to the scientific lineage into which Diana was born. Her father was the founding chair of the computer science department at Stanford University, and her equally brilliant mother—while denied the opportunities that Diana's father had enjoyed—nevertheless played a similar founding role in computer science education. In a scientific family Diana's decision to become an anthropologist in some ways made her the anomaly, but in other ways she carried on family traditions. As she mentions in the essay "George and Sandra's Daughter, Robert's Girl," her family's Quaker heritage set for her a standard of intellectual integrity. Indeed, the phrase "to speak truth to power" that she describes as characteristic of her mother's integrity also could be taken as a theme of her work.

Diana received her bachelor's degree in anthropology and sociology from Swarthmore College in 1969. She did her dissertation fieldwork in Scotland, received her doctorate in cultural anthropology and social demography from Cornell University in 1974, and served as an assistant professor of anthropology at the University of Wisconsin, Appleton. She subsequently did fieldwork in Germany, where she lived in 1976–78 and again in 1981–85. Her contributions to European studies included publications on urban-rural migration and studies of rural education. She served as a visiting lecturer or research fellow at Oxford University, the University of Bielefeld, the University of Cologne, and the University of Aberdeen.

In 1985 Diana returned to the United States and moved to her hometown of Palo Alto. Upon attending a twentieth-anniversary celebration of Stanford's computer science department, she was invited to visit the lab of a researcher who had known her father. The visit inaugurated a career change that eventually led to the influential essays that are collected in this volume. In 1987–88 Diana completed postdoctoral study in artificial intelligence (AI) at Stanford University, and she subsequently became a research scientist in the Department of Computer Science at the University of Pittsburgh. There she also served as an associate of the Center for Medical Ethics and a fellow of the Center for Philosophy of Science. In 1992 she was promoted to research associate professor, and in 1994 she became a visiting scholar in the Program in Science, Technology, and Society at Stanford University. She subsequently became an associate adjunct professor in the Medical Anthropology Program, Department of Epidemiology and Biostatistics, at the University of California at San Francisco.

During the course of her career, Diana received many awards and honors, and she played a leadership role in the professional societies to which she belonged. She received funding from several prestigious organizations, including the National Institutes of Health, the British Social Science Research Council, and the U.S. National Library of Medicine. She was elected a fellow of both the Royal Anthropological Institute and the Association of Social Anthropologists of Great Britain. She worked as an editorial board member of the official journal of the Society for Social Studies of Science (*Science, Technology, and Human Values*) and of the journal *Machine-Mediated Learning*. A special issue of *Science, Technology, and Human Values* on "Anthropological Approaches in Science and Technology Studies" (Layne 1998) is dedicated to her memory, and an issue of the *Anthropology of Work Review*

(Hogle and Downey 1999) is dedicated to articles that develop ideas in her paper "Ethics and Politics of Studying Up."

Diana had played a key role in bringing together various groups of anthropologists to form the Committee on the Anthropology of Science, Technology, and Computing of the General Anthropology Division of the American Anthropological Association. The committee, also known as CASTAC, became the institutional locus for the emerging subfield in the United States. Through her position as program chair of the Society for the Anthropology of Work and' as council member of the Society for Social Studies of Science, Diana was developing working relationships among the various subfields of anthropology and building relationships between anthropologists and the general science and technology studies community. Always friendly and known for her kindness, she was a key and irreplaceable person in a growing network of researchers. Many of us considered her both a friend and colleague.

OVERVIEW

This volume draws together Diana's unpublished papers in the anthropology of science and technology plus some of her published research that helps reveal the trajectory of her thinking. Organized in roughly chronological order, the chapters chart the main lines of her research in the 1980s and 1990s. They focus on problems in what were formerly known as expert systems, that is, computer-based information systems that were developed within the subfield of computer science known as AI research. Expert or knowledge-based systems were originally conceptualized as replacements for, not aids for, experts' knowledge. Due to the kinds of failures that Diana documents in this volume, the systems gradually evolved into a more supplementary role for expert knowledge. An example is a system that answers the questions of patients about a disease or that helps physicians to make diagnoses.

Diana did extensive fieldwork in medical informatics and AI during the 1980s and 1990s, working in four knowledge-based systems laboratories in academia and one in industry for a period of about eight years. In order to appreciate better what Diana was up against when she spoke clearly and honestly as an anthropologist, it is important to understand the position of AI during the 1980s, when she began fieldwork. During this period AI enjoyed a highly privileged position both in the worlds of computer science and in the privileged worlds of defense funding. Millions of dollars were given freely by funding agencies such as DARPA (Defense Advanced Research Projects Agency) or ONR (Office of Naval Research) to researchers in AI, especially at elite schools such as Stanford, Carnegie-Mellon, and MIT. Very often the supported projects were "blue-sky," that is, unconstrained by deliverable technology or any rigors of development. Under this aegis, many AI researchers were able to enjoy a freedom to range in their questioning across psychology, linguistics, history of science, philosophy, and biology, to name a few disciplines. Some researchers even took a kind of pride in "never writing a line of code," as evidence of their status as pure thinkers.

Such an atmosphere made Diana's task even more challenging. The delicate act of "studying up," while respecting both one's own and others' points of view, was compounded by the rarefied atmosphere in AI at the time. Restoring the work and the context, as Diana did with courage, required that she speak about unpopular topics such as getting one's hands dirty in the practice of work or acknowledging the historical specificity of the discoveries and frameworks that were emerging from the field. She did this work before the emergence of a more widespread development of a community of social scientists working in and alongside computer scientists—a lonely voyage, indeed.

As a result of her long fieldwork exposure, Diana gradually developed a profound understanding of the culture of AI research. With that understanding came an analysis of how the assumptions of AI researchers limit their horizons of understanding and lead to problems with the systems they build. The first three chapters—"Blaming the User in Medical Informatics," "The Construction of Work in Artificial Intelligence," and "Engineering Knowledge"—form an interrelated group that explores some of the reasons for the failure of knowledge-based systems. In the first chapter Diana examines one problem with the systems: users sometimes become frustrated with the systems and leave them on the shelves. AI researchers tend to refer to the problem as "the problem of user acceptance," and they explain this "end-user failure" as the result of computer-phobia or other types of shortcomings on the part of their customers. In other words, they blame the user, not themselves, for the failure.

In contrast to the blame-the-user viewpoint, Diana examines how the culture of AI researchers creates limitations in the design of knowledge-based systems. To begin, she argues that AI researchers have a culture, which she defines in terms of the taken-for-granted in social life. As in other scientific communities, AI researchers tend to think that they do not have a culture. They are instead "purely" technical. Diana insists that the technical is itself cultural and, furthermore, that AI researchers have a special kind of technical culture that is characterized by features such as technical bias; decontextualized thinking; quantitative, formal bias (seen especially in the use of clinical trials for evaluation methods); a preference for explicit models; and a tendency to believe that there is only one correct interpretation (or reality) of events.

The second essay, "The Construction of Work in Artificial Intelligence," continues and deepens Diana's analysis of the culture of AI researchers. Taking "work" as a native category, she examines what work means to AI researchers. Although, as mentioned above, some elite researchers may take pride in not writing code, Diana finds that for most AI researchers writing code tends to be a central part of the definition of what "work" means in the AI culture. However, as she spent time among the AI researchers, she realized that writing code was actually a very small percentage of all the different tasks that they perform. The head of her laboratory even pointed out that he had not written code for a decade. The narrowness of the conception of work corresponds to the narrowness and brittleness of the systems that knowledge engineers build. To invoke a phrase that Diana develops in this chapter, the systems tend to "fall off the knowledge cliff"; that is, they give patently absurd answers. One example involved a diagnosis of a bacterial infection in a male patient; the system suggested that he might have had prior amniocentesis. In a foreshadowing of her subsequent essays, Diana explores why no one thought to include a commonsense rule about the gender of the patient in the diagnostic system.

In the third chapter, "Engineering Knowledge," Diana explores the parallel problem of how AI researchers define knowledge, which they divide into expertise and common sense. In general, knowledge engineers tend to focus on explicit, technical knowledge and expertise, which lends itself relatively easily to the formal rules that they can encode in their systems. Their methods for eliciting knowledge for their expert systems also tend to be formal and to focus on conscious or explicit models of technical knowledge. In all aspects of the culture of AI—their understandings and practices related to work, knowledge, methods for building systems, methods for evaluating the systems, and explanations for why systems fail—Diana argues that knowledge engineers tend to "delete the social," a concept that she borrows from her colleague Leigh Star (1991) and that she develops in other essays. The result is that knowledge engineers tend to produce artificial knowledges that are static, brittle, and narrow.

In her explication of the culture of AI and its implications for expert system design, Diana uses as a point of comparison her own training in interpretive anthropology and her use of ethnographic fieldwork as a knowledge elicitation method. Thus, her work takes on a complex, reflexive dimension that is revealed through an exchange that followed publication of "Engineering Knowledge" in *Social Studies of Science*. The article and exchange have an interesting publication story that those of us who were close to Diana had heard from her. The editor of *Social Studies of Science*, David Edge, has a reputation for helping researchers publish their first articles in the science and technology studies (STS) literature. He heard Diana give the paper "Engineering Knowledge" in 1987, and he requested that she send him a copy. She did so and eventually submitted a revised version for publication. The three reviewers had all done empirical studies of AI, but none was an anthropologist. From Diana's files we know that one of the reviewers was the management and policy researcher James Fleck, whose objections were eventually published in the exchange included here. Because the other two reviewers were split on the extent of revision that was needed, Edge returned the paper and informed Diana that it would have to be revised and resubmitted.

Somewhat later another paper arrived at the journal, and an associate editor sent it to Diana for review. Because the paper had very different theoretical assumptions from her own, Diana refused to review it and asked the editor to send it to a reviewer who was more comfortable with its theoretical assumptions. She saw the issue as one of academic fairness, and it is an example of her strong sense of academic integrity. She also suggested that as an "experiment" a revised version of her paper be reviewed by anthropologists. The editor, to his credit, accepted her suggestions. The two anthropologists who reviewed the paper gave it high praise (indeed, I was one of them). According to Diana's notes, the third reviewer, Fleck, sent a photocopy of his first review. He highlighted passages that in his view were still in need of attention. Apparently the differences were substantial enough that, in his view, his fundamental objections had not been answered by the revised version. As Edge commented, "Our judgment was that the differences between Diana's and Jamie's positions were sufficiently and interestingly distinct to justify a public exchange between them" (personal correspondence to Hess, November 1998). Whereas Diana thought that publication of only the negative review unfairly biased readers against her paper, Edge did not want to devote space to reviewers who essentially were in agreement with her. The background on the publication history should help readers to understand the exchange in its immediate context.

Fleck begins his commentary by acknowledging that Diana's approach would improve the work of knowledge engineers. However, he then accuses her of "unequivocally saying that the social scientists' view is *right*," a position that he rejects as "epistemologically asymmetric" (1994: 106). He charges that Diana's asymmetric stance forecloses the possibility of reflexively using the work of knowledge engineers to question social scientists. Furthermore, he accuses her of stereotyping knowledge engineers through a patronizing analysis that is similar to racism. He also criticizes Diana's use of Star's concept of the "deletion of the social" (1991) because it had "negative overtones" (1994: 109). Instead, he suggests that engineers "do not so much wantonly destroy the social, as *inflate* the technical" (1994: 109). In turn, he charges Diana with deleting the technical.

Diana was troubled by Fleck's criticism, and as several of us who knew her remember well, she worked carefully to craft her reply. She begins her reply by noting that Fleck's "positivist" orientation contrasts with her own cultural relativism, and the result is a communicative impasse. She writes, "Statements about paradigmatic differences strike the [positivist] as a put-down, whereas to the relativist they constitute simple description" (1994: 114). Consequently, she sees her exchange with Fleck as "replicat[ing] the epistemological disjunction" that was the subject of her paper (114). The disjunction allows Fleck to misread her as claiming that her anthropological perspective is superior to that of the knowledge engineers. "Rather, my point is that the epistemological stance taken by members of two particular disciplinary communities is not the same, and that such epistemological commitments have consequences for the way the members of these communities go about their work" (115).

Diana then makes some significant general comments about how she understands ethnography as an anthropologist, and in the process she helps to articulate the "second wave" of ethnographic studies of science in the STS field. In contrast to the earlier laboratory studies, which focused on philosophical issues involving the construction of knowledge and the issue of epistemological relativism, Diana's work was part of a second wave of ethnographies that was carried out largely by anthropologists and broadly interested in issues of culture and power. In her discussion of ethnographic method, Diana distinguishes between an explicit critique of cultural practices, which she sees as a legitimate anthropological task in the sense developed by George Marcus and Michael Fischer (1986), from patronizing a people, which she, like other anthropologists, deplores. She adds that Fleck's willingness to instruct her on her own discipline is "remarkable" and "reflects a certain tendency within STS to appropriate anthropology" (117). Rather than aspire to neutrality, as Fleck would have for anthropology, Diana suggests that "awareness" of one's own epistemological commitments, as well as those of one's informants, is a better goal. Furthermore, she adds that Fleck's vision of the anthropologist as a researcher who should speak for her informants is outdated, even colonialist. Instead, she defends a view of ethnography that begins with the worldview or perspectives of one's informants, the "stepping in" of ethnographic immersion, to use the phrase of anthropologist Hortense Powdermaker (1966). However, ethnography has an equally if not more important second step of critical analysis that involves "stepping out" from the informants' perspectives. In this way, Diana suggests a distinction between cultural relativism (a method) and epistemological relativism, which has plagued some wings of science studies and which Fleck seems to endorse. Indeed, she finds that her informants valued precisely the critical analysis that Fleck found problematic.

Diana's reply remains controversial to this day. Some readers have argued the issue from the opposite side of the spectrum from Fleck. For example, her colleague David Hakken writes, "For purposes of creating a workable 'expert system,' Forsythe's critique *does* lay the basis for an approach superior to that of the engineers she studies" (1999: 225). Whether one wishes to characterize the issue as when to step in versus when to step out, a theoretical balancing of cultural relativism and epistemological antirelativism, or descriptive versus normative discourse, the continued discussion of the debate in the anthropological research community suggests that it crystallizes a central tension of ethnographic work, particularly in the anthropology of science, technology, and work.

The next essay, "Artificial Intelligence Invents Itself: Collective Identity and Boundary Maintenance in an Emergent Scientific Discipline," is concerned with the question of boundaries, although not the kinds of social science boundaries that characterized the Fleck–Forsythe exchange. The paper was filed as a report with the Computer Science Department at the University of Pittsburgh, where Diana worked, and, although less well known than her published essays, deserves to have wider circulation. The essay examines the question of boundaries both within AI as a community and between AI and other academic fields. Diana describes an orthodox view of AI as an experimental, hard science that studies intelligence, but she also finds dissenting views that maintain, for example, that AI is "just software engineering." She also explores the tacit meanings involved in boundary-making statements, such as the claim that something is "not AI." As a whole, the essay provides a deeper exploration of the culture of AI, both in terms of how it is defined in opposition to its Others, and in terms of how orthodox and heterodox currents of AI produce tensions within the research community.

The next essay included here, "New Bottles, Old Wine," involves the design of an expert system that would educate migraine patients. In this case, Diana's research program deepens as she helps to write a proposal and serves as a coinvestigator in a project that includes a role for her vision of ethnography in the construction of an expert system. One might expect that the innovative project would result in the construction of a better system, but her work became marginalized. What happened? In a postmortem analysis, she shows that the AI designers began with the expert knowledge of the physicians, and the anthropologists recorded the often tacit knowledge of the physicians and the patients. Unfortunately, as Diana writes, "The ethnographic material was inconsistent with design elements to which they had committed in the early stages of conventional knowledge acquisition with the physician-expert." In principle it would still be possible for ethnographic knowledge to play a greater role in the design of expert systems, but the whole process of collaboration would have to be rethought from the starting point, and that would mean altering significantly the power relations between the AI researchers and the social scientists on the team.

Diana's analysis brings out an important consequence of the failure to incorporate ethnographic analysis into system design. The loss of ethnographic analysis corresponds to the loss of the knowledge, needs, and perspectives of patients. The point deserves emphasis because it reveals another aspect of the analysis that was missing in Fleck's critique. There are actually several informant communities in question—AI researchers, the experts (physicians in this case), and the users, who in the case of medical informatics are laypersons and/or patients. The work of the AI researchers tends to select the voices of the experts and ignore or marginalize those of the patients. That the experts and AI researchers tend to be privileged males, and the patients tend to be more diverse in terms of status and gender, was a point that Diana did not miss. Although her feminist analysis is somewhat compressed in this essay, she flagged the issue here. In other words, understandings of knowledge and knowledge elicitation methods are gendered. In this case a woman anthropologist worked with male knowledge engineers who encoded the knowledge of male experts for use by what often turned out to be female patients. As she explained to those of us who knew her, she tended to downplay the analysis of gender in her essays of the early 1990s because she did not want to offend her informants and employers.

Diana analyzed the problem of her positionality in her essay "Ethics and Politics of Studying Up in Technoscience." The paper later became the topic of a memorial session, which was organized by her colleagues for the 1998 annual meeting of the American Anthropological Association and subsequently published in the volume of the *Anthropology of Work Review* mentioned earlier (Hogle and Downey 1999). As with many women in science, including her mother, Diana had a nontraditional career. She did not have a tenured position that would have been appropriate for the many awards, publications, grants, academic appointments, and fieldwork projects on her CV. Instead, until 1994 she worked on soft money as the resident ethnographer in AI laboratories. Not only did she lack the protections and the prestige of tenure, but she had to work as a woman in a world of men. As has occurred increasingly with anthropologists since the 1960s, her work violated almost all of the assumptions of the traditional fieldwork narrative of the anthropologist who goes off to a foreign country to live among poor people in a rural village. Instead, her informants were her employers; they even had veto power over her publication. As many of us have found when working with well-educated informants, they care very much about how they are quoted and portrayed in print, and we often have to give some ground to those considerations to avoid litigation or to retain access. As anthropologists continue to work in increasing numbers with well-educated, powerful communities, they face new risks, both for themselves and for their informants. Diana's case is exemplary because its extreme nature led to difficult ethical dilemmas. For example, she was caught between wanting to help her informants and being positioned institutionally as their competitor for scarce resources in the laboratory. She also became involved in a controversy over the ownership of her fieldwork data, and the university lawyers ruled against her. The event was shocking to many of her colleagues in anthropology, where fieldwork notes are regarded as private (often highly private) property.

In the next two essays, "Studying Those Who Study Us" and "It's Just a Matter of Common Sense," Diana takes up the next phase of the problem. She proposed that, in effect, she and other ethnographers of computer-mediated design had won the battle but lost the war. As the expert systems segment of the medical informatics community had begun to accept the basic argument that social science perspectives and methods, especially ethnography, could be useful in computer-mediated design projects, knowledge engineers tended to appropriate ethnography for themselves. The result was, to continue Star's metaphor, that they deleted the ethnographer. In an ironic turn of events, Diana recalls attending a medical informatics meeting in which researchers with no training in ethnography or anthropology presented "ethnographic" research. One was a physician who was inspired to try ethnography after reading her papers. Although the story is amusing, Diana points out in "Studying Those Who Study Us" that the phenomenon carries with it problematic disciplinary power dimensions. For example, AI ethnographers had become competitors with anthropologists for federal funding for social science research.

The politics of positionality that Diana discusses are also embedded in the twin papers. "Studying Those Who Study Us" is clearly written for anthropologists, and it was presented at the annual meeting of the American Anthropological Association. In contrast, "It's Just a Matter of Common Sense" was published in *Computer Supported Cooperative Work* in a special issue on the "structure of invisible work" edited by Bonnie Nardi and Yrjö Engeström (1999). Although the two papers overlap, we have decided to publish them both here, partly because their differences of emphasis reveal the ways in which anthropologists of science negotiate their membership in their home and field communities.

Both articles mention a complaint that those of us who knew Diana remember her making on occasion. People in the AI community sometimes came to her and said, "I'd like to do some ethnography for my expert system. Can you give me an article I can read over the weekend to teach me how to do it?" To her the request was absurd. It would be similar to a layperson coming to a surgeon and asking to borrow a book to learn how to do surgery over the weekend. Her point was that the ability to do good ethnography requires a lengthy training and practice; the training includes reading a great deal of social science theory as well as many exemplary ethnographies, and then having long periods of actual fieldwork experience. Indeed, for most cultural or social anthropologists, learning to do good ethnography is at the core of their five or more years of graduate training.

Diana was therefore grappling with what might be called culture change in the AI community: the emergence of "do-it-yourself" ethnography. While new, the phenomenon also represented a selection and reconstruction of ethnography as it became part of AI culture. As Diana explains the differences between her own assumptions about ethnography and those held by AI researchers, she also develops a very thoughtful description of ethnographic research methods—perhaps the best to emerge to date in the anthropology of science, technology, and work. One of the key distinctions—which occurs with many other disciplines that claim to be using ethnography—is that the long-term experience that Diana has accumulated as an ethnographer (years of work in several laboratories) is collapsed into short-term interviews or observation. Yet even with short-term studies, Diana finds that the AI researchers do relatively little with the data, largely because their frameworks tend to take local meanings at face value and to overlook tacit meanings. As she comments in "Studying Those Who Study Us":

> Since the powerful "old boys" of medical informatics have not always welcomed critique of their assumptions, the absence of a critical edge in this "insider" ethnography probably makes it much more palatable from their standpoint. While this work may add little in terms of new understanding, it also does not rock the boat—something to which the old boys are rather sensitive.

The final two essays address explicitly the issues of gender, power, and feminism that implicitly informed Diana's work from the beginning. When delivered at conferences, the papers generated a great deal of enthusiasm from her colleagues, who were encouraging her to develop the topic before she met with her untimely death. In "Disappearing Women in the Social World of Computing," Diana continues the "deletion-of-the-social/cultural" theme that traversed her work, focusing now on the deletion of women and gender from the culture of AI research. The process occurs on multiple levels.

To begin, there is the "pipeline" problem of few women professionals in the field, a problem that Diana links to her memories of her mother's exclusion from a career in the field. Beyond the pipeline problem, the culture of AI tends to "disappear" those women who are there. Diana keenly reviews some of the mechanisms through which the disappearances occur. For example, she documents an instance of sexual harassment that appears non-gendered to the lab workers because the men interpret the act as a non-gendered practical joke. Next, Diana revisits the construction of work issue and argues that because most of the women in the labs do administrative or staff work, their work is not considered important or "real" work. As a result, statements such as "there are no women in the lab" become possible, even when they are made in front of women workers. The process of ignoring women is linked to the tendency to ignore degrees other than the M.D., including the Ph.D. and degrees such as an R.N. or M.L.S., which many of the women hold. Even women's bodies tend to be deleted. For example, Diana describes a man who ignores a woman's obviously pregnant body because he is not sure whether she has gained weight or is indeed pregnant. Finally, Diana shows how women in the AI community participate in their own disappearing act. In one of her classic examples of speaking truth to power, Diana writes, "I speculate that the prevailing tacit deletion of women and gender issues, plus the gendered power hierarchy in computer fields, may combine to pressure women either to join in the silence or to leave the field." She suggests that it would be interesting to carry out exit interviews with women who have left the field. Likewise, she suggests that her analysis has policy implications that reveal the problem of chronically low (and dropping) participation of women in computer science to be a cultural issue as much as a "pipeline issue."

The final essay of this volume is the most personal. Here Diana discusses "kinship" in science, both in the sense of the personal networks among scientists and their staffs and in the sense of her family relations. To begin with the former, the essay develops the concept of the laboratory as a kind of fictive kin group, thus extending her anthropological analysis to a concept that could be generally important to other anthropologists working in laboratory settings. As a kin-like unit, the laboratory head (usually an older male) encompasses the laboratory members. For example, Diana became known to members of other labs as "Robert's girl." Likewise, the labs are related to each other through their leaders, and social relationships among researchers are defined with respect to membership in laboratories. The fictive kin identification that Diana held as "Robert's girl" or "Robert's anthropologist" therefore gave her a position in the world of AI, and it served to keep her from becoming completely invisible when speaking with men from other laboratories. At the same time, the identification positioned her in a logic of gendered, disciplinary, and generational supplementarity that was similar to the relations in the household in which she grew up. Her father had become a famous computer scientist and her mother, also a brilliant scientist, had suffered from marginalization. Although very serious in import, the essay also reveals moments of Diana's characteristic (and feminist) humor, such as her self-characterization as a "computer science princess."

The tragedy of premature death is a theme that runs through the last essay of the book—the death of Marianne Paget, an accomplished medical sociologist; of Diana's father, whose life she was exploring by going through his archived documents at Stanford shortly before her own untimely death; and her mother, whose life in many ways Diana had come to see as a mirror for her own. At one level the essay was a personal attempt to come to terms with the tragedy of her parents' premature deaths. (Her mother's brother also died prematurely, from a drowning accident at age seventeen.) At the same time, she was puzzling through the implications of the opposing fates of her father and mother. Whereas her father was remembered (having a building, computer system, and lecture named after him), her mother—also an important figure in the history of computer science due to her work in computer education—faced systematic sex discrimination and has been all but forgotten.

Like her parents, Diana was a founding member of a new field—in this case the anthropology of science and technology and its intersection with the anthropology of work and feminist anthropology—and she suffered a sudden death that, as she says of her father, curtailed her plans and dreams. Anthropologists are now working to ensure that Diana's memory is not deleted from the disciplinary consciousness, and this book represents a step toward preserving her legacy.

—David J. Hess
*Rensselaer Polytechnic Institute*

Diana had planned to develop a book from her essays, and she had initiated conversations with presses, but she was unable to fulfill her dream. Although Diana probably would have rewritten the papers into a coherent whole that would have eliminated repetitions and cross-referencing, we have decided that it would be best to publish the materials in the condition in which they were found—that is, as independent essays. The editorial decision results in some minor repetitions and much cross-referencing across the chapters. Whereas some of the substantial repetitions have been deleted (and flagged in the endnotes), I have kept most of the cross-referencing.

To ensure accuracy, I started from the computer files of her papers and compared them against hard copies of the unpublished papers or reprints of the published papers. In two cases she left behind "errata" sheets, and the corrections are incorporated here. For unpublished papers I have used the most recent version available. Endnotes have been altered in some cases to correspond with the name-and-date citation system, but no substantive material was deleted.

The introduction and selection of essays is a collaborative project undertaken by several of Diana's colleagues. I would like to thank Gary Downey, Joe Dumit, David Hakken, Linda Layne, Bonnie Nardi, John Singleton, Lucy Suchman, Leigh Star, and Chris Toumey for their support and comments on the project as a whole and Nicki Dusyk for proofreading a final version of the edited manuscript. They and the press's reviewers and editors provided helpful criticisms and wording additions and deletions for the introductory essay. Some of the colleagues also wrote obituaries that appeared in *Social Studies of Science*, 1998, 28 (1): 175–82. Diana's widower, Bern Shen, was instrumental in finding the unpublished articles and digital files, securing permissions, and otherwise helping the publication process to completion. Chris

Toumey organized a memorial panel at the American Anthropological Association, which provided an occasion to discuss the book project.

"Blaming the User in Medical Informatics: The Cultural Nature of Scientific Practice" was published in *Knowledge and Society, Vol. 9: The Anthropology of Science and Technology*, ed. by David Hess and Linda Layne, 1992, 9: 95–111, and is reprinted here with permission from JAI Press.

"The Construction of Work in Artificial Intelligence" was published in *Science, Technology, and Human Values*, 1993, 18: 460–79, and is reprinted here with permission from Sage Publications, Inc.

"Engineering Knowledge: The Construction of Knowledge in Artificial Intelligence," "Knowing Engineers?: A Response to Forsythe" (by James Fleck), and "STS (Re)constructs Anthropology: A Reply to Fleck" were published in *Social Studies of Science* (respectively, 1993, 23: 445–77; 1994, 24: 105–13; and 1994, 24: 113–23) and are reprinted here with permission from Sage Publications, Inc.

"Artificial Intelligence Invents Itself" was first presented at the 1988 meeting of the Society for Social Studies of Science and was published as the Report No. ISL-90-8 and CS-90-8 of the Intelligent Systems Laboratory, Computer Science Department, University of Pittsburgh. It is reprinted here with permission.

"New Bottles, Old Wine: Hidden Cultural Assumptions in a Computerized Explanation System for Migraine Sufferers" was published in *Medical Anthropology Quarterly*, 1996, 10 (4): 551–74, and is reprinted here with permission from Bern Shen.

"Ethics and Politics of Studying Up in Technoscience" was presented at the 1995 annual meeting of the American Anthropological Association, Washington, D.C.; revised on November 5, 1996; and published posthumously in the *Anthropology of Work Review*, 1999, 20 (1): 6–11, and it is reprinted here with permission from Bern Shen.

"Studying Those Who Study Us: Medical Informatics Appropriates Ethnography" was presented at the 1996 annual meeting of the American Anthropological Association, San Francisco, and revised on March 21, 1997. Both are published here with permission from Bern Shen.

"'It's Just a Matter of Common Sense': Ethnography as Invisible Work" was published in *Computer-Supported Cooperative Work*, 1998, 1–2: 127–45, in a special issue coedited by Bonnie Nardi and Yrjö Engeström titled "A Web on the Wind: The Structure of Invisible Work." The essay is reprinted here with permission from Kluwer, Inc.

"Disappearing Women in the Social World of Computing" was presented at the 1994 meeting of the American Anthropological Association, Atlanta, and revised on May 2, 1996; and "George and Sandra's Daughter, Robert's Girl: Doing Ethnographic Research in My Parents' Field" was presented at the 1997 meeting of the American Ethnological Society, Seattle, and revised on March 21, 1997. Both are published with permission from Bern Shen.

Royalties from this project will go to the Diana Forsythe Prize, offered jointly by the Committee for the Anthropology of Science, Technology, and Computing (CASTAC) and the Society for the Anthropology of Work of the American Anthropological Association. To make donations, please contact the association in Arlington, Virginia.

# CHAPTER ONE

# Blaming the User in Medical Informatics: The Cultural Nature of Scientific Practice

This paper is a report from a long-term project on styles of thought and action in artificial intelligence (AI) (see chs. 2, 3, 6).[1] The investigation focuses upon the relationship among the values and assumptions that a community of scientists bring to their work; the actions that constitute that work; and the tools they construct in the course of that work.[2] My informants are members of the expert systems community within AI, and their tools are the complex computer programs known as knowledge-based or expert systems.

The values and assumptions shared within a group constitute part of what anthropologists call "culture." Culture defines what we take for granted, including explicit, formal truths of the sort embodied in scientific paradigms; the tacit values and assumptions that underlie formal theory; and the common sense truths that "everybody knows" within a given setting (or type of setting). Our cultural background thus influences the way in which we make sense of particular situations, as well as the actions perceived as possible and meaningful in any given situation (Geertz 1973, 1983).

In other papers I discuss the central concepts of "knowledge," "work," and "information" in AI, examining the relation between my informants' understanding of these notions and the way they go about their work (see chs. 2, 3, and Forsythe, Buchanan, Osheroff, and Miller 1992). In so doing, I have explicitly argued that their scientific practice is cultural. This is not meant to imply that my informants' way of construing the world is totally different from that of their colleagues in other countries, people in other academic disciplines, or Americans in general. On the contrary, in all three cases one would expect to find a good deal in common; thus, it would be inaccurate to speak of a discrete "culture of artificial intelligence." Instead, what I assert is that people who are accepted as belonging to the AI community share *some* meanings and practices with each other that they do not necessarily share with other people. Being seen to share these is an important criterion of membership in this community. In order to understand what these individuals are doing when they "do science" as they define it, we need to understand what these shared meanings and practices are.

The anthropologist's assertion that science is cultural is not intuitively obvious to the scientists with whom we work. For example, my informants' understanding of their own work as "hard science" means to them that they are part of a universal truth-seeking enterprise that is above or outside of culture (chs. 3, 6). Nor is this cultural perspective necessarily shared by other outside observers who question this positivist view of science. In examining decisions about what is taken to be true in science, social scientists often focus upon the social construction of scientific truth while largely avoiding the issue of the cultural contexts within which such construction takes place. Thus, for example, a growing body of research analyzes the social and rhetorical devices that scientists use to construct problems as doable (Fujimura 1987), findings as visible (Knorr-Cetina and Amann 1990), and particular technologies as "the right tool(s) for the job" (Clarke and Casper 1991, Clarke and Fujimura 1992). Detailed local-level (Lynch 1985, Latour and Woolgar 1986) and broader (Latour 1987, Collins 1985) studies have illuminated the negotiations and power struggles that underlie scientific outcomes. Over the past decade or so, these and many other studies have documented the socially contingent nature of science. Such studies contribute a great deal to our understanding of science and technology. However, within this growing STS literature, relatively little attention has been devoted to examining the fact that scientific processes are culturally contingent as well. This imbalance is likely to be redressed by the emerging anthropology of science and technology (Suchman 1987, Traweek 1988a, Downey 1988, Hess 1991, Pfaffenberger 1988, Hess and Layne 1992).

Perhaps because the scientists we study often come from cultural backgrounds related to our own, observers of science sometimes appear to take cultural knowledge for granted. Yet such knowledge is an important source of the concepts and interpretations used to construct scientific truths. While the beliefs held by actors within a given scientific setting or community are neither identical nor altogether stable over time, neither are they completely reinvented from one event to the next. Scientists construct local meanings and struggle to position themselves within a cultural context against a backdrop of more enduring beliefs, at least some of which competing actors hold in common. After all, in order to negotiate at all or successfully to frame actions or objects in a given light, there must be overlap in the interpretive possibilities available to the parties concerned. As scientists construct artifacts and meanings, they draw upon a repertoire of familiar beliefs about the way the world is ordered, some of which are explicit and some of which remain tacit. Among other things, such meanings embody understandings about what can be a problem and what can be a solution. An important concern of the anthropologist of science is to illuminate these beliefs and investigate their relationship to scientific practice.

In this paper, I will pursue this theme with reference to a current issue in medical informatics, one of the major application areas of AI. The issue is the so-called problem of user acceptance: the fact that medical expert systems are rarely adopted for routine use. This problem is currently a focus of concern in medical informatics and, therefore, among my informants in that field. I will argue that although they are genuinely concerned about this problem and appear to be baffled by it, their own procedures are in a sense causing the difficulty. That is, the problem of user acceptance is to a significant extent the outcome of values and assumptions that the scientists bring to their own research and development process. While I do not suggest that this connection is conscious or intentional, the nature of this particular tradition of scientific practice makes it very difficult for its followers to see or entertain research strategies from other traditions that would probably help to solve their problem.

## BACKGROUND

Medical informatics involves the application of computer science, information science, and intelligent systems technology to problems in medicine. It is a relatively new field: the first medical expert systems were built in the 1970s, and the first textbook on the subject appeared in 1990 (Shortliffe, Perreault, Wiederhold, and Fagan 1990). General acceptance of "medical informatics" as the name of this field has only occurred within the past two or three years, as that term has displaced the names "medical computer science," "medical information science," and "artificial intelligence and medicine" as the term by which practitioners identify their field. Since the mid-seventies, the major funding for medical informatics has come from a single non-military government funding agency, which supports research, infrastructure, and a number of post-graduate training programs at major American universities. The products of these training programs, almost exclusively white men, generally emerge with both an M.D. and a Ph.D., enabling them eventually to attain positions of considerable power in the world of academic medicine.

## The Field Study

Since 1986, I have been a full-time participant-observer in a series of AI laboratories. Four of these are academic labs; two are exclusively concerned with medical expert systems, and the other two produce both medical and non-medical systems. (A fifth lab, in which I spent only a few weeks, is a commercial lab that produces no medical systems.) Thus, most of my participant-observation has involved the world of medical informatics. Since 1988, I have been funded exclusively from projects in medical informatics. In addition to ongoing participant-observation in AI labs, I have in connection with these projects taken part in numerous meetings with representatives of funding agencies, in national conferences, and in writing teams that have produced several proposals and publications in the field. For these projects, I have also carried out some short-term fieldwork in medical settings.

In moving thus in and out of a range of laboratory and other professional settings in AI and medical informatics, I have attempted to study a scientific community rather than to focus exclusively upon one or more laboratories as bounded social entities. This community-centered approach to the study of science and technology follows that developed by Traweek (1988a), extending the laboratory-centered approach adopted by Latour and Woolgar (1986), Knorr-Cetina (1981), and Lynch (1985).

## The Problem of User Acceptance

The American College of Medical Informatics (ACMI) is an elected body of leaders in the field. In 1991, ACMI met to discuss the direction of medical informatics for the 1990s.[3] They produced a list of problems facing the field, a list intended to guide research during the coming decade. First on the list was the problem of user acceptance.

While medical informatics has been producing intelligent systems for medical settings for nearly twenty years, these systems have not been widely adopted for daily use. In fact, one senior member of the field estimated that fewer than ten such systems are in actual routine use—and that number includes systems used by one doctor in one site a few times per week. A junior colleague put the matter even more pessimistically. Asked what had happened to all the systems produced over the years, he replied, "They're all on the shelf." To understand how this can be the case, we turn now to a consideration of some of the shared assumptions and work practices characteristic of medical informatics.

## STANDARD OPERATING PROCEDURE IN MEDICAL INFORMATICS

In medical informatics, it is widely accepted that physicians suffer from major problems involving information access, management, and transmission. This is known as the problem of physicians' information needs. It is also widely accepted that this problem can only be mastered through the use of automation. Taken together, these beliefs form the charter for medical informatics, whose practitioners design and build complex computer systems intended to support information access and management in medicine. Given the obvious truth of these beliefs from the perspective of specialists in medical informatics, the problem of user acceptance is understandably baffling. If physicians need these systems so much, why don't they use them?

Although the systems are intended to be useful, the unenthusiastic response in the medical community suggests that they are not perceived as such. That is, knowledge-based systems are apparently not seen as useful enough to warrant the time, trouble, and expense of using them. Clearly, something is wrong: to borrow a commonplace from software engineering, it would seem that either medical informatics is not building the right systems or it is not building the systems right. When my informants are asked to account for this, they tend to blame the users. One designer asserted that "All members of the public are computerphobic." Others suggest that naive users do not know how to use the systems correctly, get frustrated, and give up—implying that these systems work fine if you know how to use them. From the designers' side, then, it would seem that if anyone is to blame for the problem of user acceptance, it is probably the users themselves. This attitude is implied by the name generally adopted for this issue: the problem of user acceptance, as opposed to, say, the problem of unusable systems. Even more straightforward is an alternative term for this problem that is also used in medical informatics: "end-user failure" (Shields, Graves, and Nyce 1991: 196).

As an outside observer, I have a different perspective on the source of this problem. Medical information systems are not being accepted because they do not meet the needs of consumers; and that difficulty in turn results from the way in which problem formulation, system design, system building, and evaluation are understood and carried out in medical informatics. To explain this, I will briefly describe some assumptions and practices that are standard in the field. They have a good deal in common with procedures accepted throughout the expert systems community, which I have described in more detail elsewhere (chs. 2, 3, 6; Forsythe and Buchanan 1989, 1991).

Problem formulation involves assessing just what a prospective system should do; once a problem is identified, a system is designed to help solve it. It is not customary—indeed, it is almost unheard of—for a design team in medical informatics to observe real-life problem-solving in the workplace in which a prospective system is intended to be fielded. Rather, design proceeds on the basis of what designers and/or experts "know" about such sites in general, that is, on the basis of their conscious models of particular types of work as carried out in particular types of settings. Thus, problem formulation and design rely heavily on intuition and introspection on the part of the system designer. In the case of designers not trained in medicine, problem formulation depends on intuition and introspection on the part of the medical expert with whom the designer is working.[4] (As in much of AI, it is customary for a design team to work with a single expert whose perspective is taken as representative of an entire field (see ch. 3). The resultant systems reflect "what everybody knows" (that is, what is taken for granted by practitioners) about tasks, settings, etc., rather than specific data on individuals actually encountering the problem that the prospective system is intended to solve. It is by no means unusual for systems to be built by designers for settings that they have never seen. For example, one AI specialist built a system intended to support a particular hospital-based branch of medicine, working in collaboration with a physician specializing in that field. When I asked whether the designer had actually visited the hospital site for which the system was intended, the astonished response was, "Oh no! I can't stand the sight of blood."

Once a system (or system prototype) has been constructed, it is refined through an iterative procedure that involves some type of evaluation. In medical informatics, evaluation tends to follow the paradigm of randomized, controlled clinical trials (CCTs) (Forsythe and Buchanan 1991). The crucial non-technical issue in evaluation is to establish whether or not the presence of a system in a particular setting affects some quantifiable behavioral variable (a so-called "outcome measure") in a statistically significant way. In evaluating a patient education system, for example, one design team decided to measure whether use of the system increased patient compliance. The evaluation design did not include investigating the patients' feelings about the system or eliciting their suggestions for improvement in the explanations it offered, nor did the team decide to observe patients actually using the system. In short, systems are evaluated and judged successful without regard to whether real-life users find them to be useful. After all, as one scientist pointed out, usefulness is not quantifiable.

From an anthropological standpoint, the CCT model is strikingly inappropriate as a model for the evaluation of a computer system. Controlled clinical trials are used for the evaluation of drug treatments, but in software evaluation the users' conscious reactions to a computer system are an important determinant of whether that system will be incorporated into clinical care. One would expect evaluation procedures in medical informatics to include methods of investigating such subjective reactions. However, drug trials are set up to control for subjective perception through the use of "blinding" procedures: the CCT model explicitly *excludes* the possibility of collecting data on patients' subjective perceptions. In adapting this model to the evaluation of medical information systems, therefore, the medical informatics community has adopted an approach that largely prevents them from getting information about users.

Thus, standard operating procedure in medical informatics includes no mechanism for investigating the needs of particular workers or the specific characteristics of their workplaces, nor does it take into account user reaction in evaluating and refining a system. Aside from the beliefs of a single designated "expert," who may not actually be expert in the particular problem-solving tasks that the system is designed to perform, the needs and desires of real users play essentially no role in the design or evaluation of medical information systems. Viewed in anthropological terms, at least, it is small wonder that medical informatics has a problem of user acceptance.

## Values and Assumptions in Medical Informatics

How can we make sense of this situation? The researchers in question are bright and highly trained individuals who understand themselves as engaged in open, scientific inquiry. Furthermore, they claim to be concerned about the problem of user acceptance. Given this problem, why don't they incorporate into their standard operating procedure what to a social scientist would be an obvious strategy: systematic investigation of users' problems, needs, and desires as well as the specific work processes into which systems are intended to fit?

I believe the answer is that these researchers are committed to a set of values and assumptions that make it difficult for them to see this strategy as desirable. In medical informatics, the very assumptions that have enabled researchers to tackle certain problems productively seem also to have made it more difficult for them to deal with other problems, or other aspects of the same problems. While these assumptions are not necessarily explicit or even conscious, they exert a significant influence on the way in which practitioners approach their work. In order to clarify this, I will outline five characteristic ways of thinking that seem to be shared by these researchers, pointing out ways in which they constrain the process of system building.

### Technical Bias

The approach to problem assessment, design, and evaluation characteristic of AI and medical informatics reflects a focus on technical factors. For example, they traditionally evaluate a system largely or entirely with respect to system performance (speed, accuracy, and—rarely—extensibility) and occasionally with respect to technical aspects of architecture (logic, complexity, and exportability). While there is nothing wrong with technical evaluation, practitioners may not be aware of how much is being left out of evaluation that looks at technical factors alone. However, to a social scientist it is clear that the omission is considerable: the non-technical includes information about social and contextual issues that are crucial to the problem of user acceptance. Such non-technical issues include whether systems are compatible with users' needs and desires, and the way users understand and evaluate a system; the way the system fits into users' normal work patterns and processes as well as into the organizational structure; and the way changes caused by the system are viewed by users, designers, and managers (see ch. 2; Fafchamps 1991; Fafchamps, Young, and Tang 1991; Forsythe and Buchanan 1991, 1992; Greenbaum and Kyng 1991). When experts and knowledge engineers define what users want and need, it seems clear that things will be left out, especially non-technical features of the work and work context that designers cannot know.

## Decontextualized Thinking

Human decision-making is complex. Artificial intelligence and medical informatics have accepted the need to simplify the information represented in knowledge-based systems in order to build such systems at all. Because such simplification has become routine in the design process, however, it seems to engender habits of thought that are carried over automatically to other areas. Thus, when practitioners think about problem-solving and evaluation, they tend to restrict their concern to questions that can be addressed using simple, quantitative models.

Star has commented that computer science "deletes the social" (1991). The social is one major category of information that gets bracketed out in the simplification process described above. Developers tend to think of systems as isolated technical objects, as the instantiation of a design. They do not necessarily consider who will work with the system once it is fielded, or how that work will be accomplished. This deletion of the social is perpetuated in the conventional wisdom on evaluation. Systems are typically evaluated only in the laboratory, out of the context in which they will eventually be expected to function. Thus, evaluation does not usually include investigation of how systems fit into the everyday social and organizational contexts in which they are to be fielded.

## Quantitative, Formal Bias

The controlled clinical trials (CCT) model brings with it the tacit assumption that "science" equals "laboratory science" and that "systematic study" requires an experiment. In medical informatics, this tends to be interpreted as meaning that to be both valid and useful, procedures must be quantitative. This bias contributes to the exclusion from problem assessment, design, and evaluation procedures of phenomena that are not amenable to quantification. Social and psychological phenomena—especially when investigated in context—do not lend themselves to study using the model of controlled experimentation: real-world settings are not easily controlled. However, it is precisely the uncontrolled, spontaneous user reaction that current system-building methods are missing. At present we do not know for sure why users do not use medical information systems, in part because we know too little about the contexts in which they are fielded, about the social and personal consequences of the use of such systems, or about the motives that contribute to people's desire to use such systems.

Software design and implementation encourage a formal perspective on problems. Much of the computer science literature is highly formal, and successful programmers are frequently trained in mathematics, logic, or a physical science. Thus, it is not surprising that system designers and implementers bring a formal perspective to their task. However, while this bias may contribute to successful system building, it has costs as well—for example, in the areas of evaluation and user acceptance. Emphasis on formal rules, procedures, facts, and relations seems to make it difficult for technical specialists to see the importance of events and relations that are not institutionalized or universal, such as the perceptions of individual users or social relations in a particular type of workplace. But although a system may be designed according to generally accepted principles, it will be fielded in a particular social and political context. While the particularities of such a context are hard to characterize in formal terms, they will play a major role in determining whether or not a system is accepted in practice.

### Conscious Models Taken as Accurate Representations of the World

In medical informatics—as in AI generally—people seem to assume that their conscious models and external "reality" are isomorphic. This assumption is reflected in the practice of designing systems solely on the basis of one expert's conscious models of particular work processes: such models are apparently taken to be accurate and complete. Experienced ethnographers would be likely to doubt this assumption. But since researchers in medical informatics do not normally undertake comparisons between conscious models and visible social patterns, the completeness and accuracy of an "expert's" generalizations are generally taken for granted.

### One Reality

Artificial intelligence takes a universalistic approach to many issues, assuming that if there is a right answer to a problem, it is right in all contexts. To put it another way, designers of AI systems, like other cognitive scientists, describe problem-solving tasks in such a way as to assume that satisfactory answers exist whose correctness can be ascertained independently of the problem-solving context. One example of this assumption at work is the practice of building a system based upon the "knowledge" of only one expert, which reflects the belief that one individual's views are representative of an entire field. The assumption of one reality is too simple to be useful in relation to such complex problems as assessing whether or not a particular type of social or technological change (such as introducing a system into health care environments) is desirable in specific circumstances. A more realistic approach would acknowledge that different individuals, and individuals in different positions, can have quite different perspectives on the same event.

*Summary*

To sum up, my informants in medical informatics are positivists who conceive of their work as "hard" science. Their model of science is a strictly bounded and rather rigid one that restricts that label to experimental undertakings involving formal, quantitative analysis of factors that they perceive as technical. This model brackets out as "soft" (and therefore unscientific) such procedures as non-directive observation, qualitative analysis, and consideration of non-technical factors.[5] I have argued that the narrowness of this notion of science, along with the assumptions upon which it rests, contribute substantially to the problem of user acceptance. Medical expert systems are built and evaluated within a narrow conceptual world. Since designers do not routinely visit work sites or talk to users, they are unlikely to come across information that would cast doubt on the generalized beliefs about work and users on which their systems are based. Lacking such data—and excluding as unscientific the informal, local information that could help them to design systems better suited to real users in particular workplaces—it is little wonder that these scientists produce systems that users do not want to use.

DISCUSSION

For purposes of discussion, I will relate this material briefly to the broader themes of culture and power. As I pointed out in the introduction, it would be inappropriate to speak of a discrete culture of medical informatics. Whether or not it makes sense to treat any human community as possessing a unique, cleanly bounded set of meanings, it does not make sense to treat medical informatics in this way. Actors in this interdisciplinary academic community belong as well to other social worlds, including other professional communities. Many of the beliefs that my informants manifest in the context of medical informatics are doubtless carried over into these other professional contexts, as well as into non-scientific contexts arising from their membership in a wider society. Setting aside the notion that medical informatics itself defines an entire culture, then, my point is that members of this field hold some beliefs and assumptions in common, and that these shared (or at least familiar) meanings relate to their scientific practice in a way that is cultural. That is, such meanings are available as a reservoir of ideas about what constitute meaningful problems and appropriate solutions in the context of medical informatics. Systems are built according to procedures that reflect these ideas, which are thereby encoded in the systems themselves (chs. 2, 3).[6]

This is not to suggest that everyone in medical informatics shares an identical set of meanings, nor that those that are shared actually determine scientific practice. After all, system-building procedures vary, scientists can and do innovate, and there is ongoing debate on such topics as what constitutes an adequate system evaluation. Rather, common values serve to frame the space within which accepted practice varies and allowable debate takes place. Thus, for example, the different methods of building and evaluating systems in what is considered mainline medical informatics *all* delete the social (chs. 2, 3, 6). Not to do so in this context is considered radical. To challenge the values that underlie accepted practice—for instance, to attempt to build and evaluate systems in a way that does not delete the social—is to run the risk of being branded a "loose cannon" and marginalized.[7]

Turning now to the second issue, I will consider two aspects of power. First, it is well known that commitment to a particular paradigm confers considerable conceptual power upon the values and assumptions that it embodies (Kuhn 1970). The case of medical informatics illustrates the cost this can have for scientists faced with a problem for which their paradigm offers few appropriate solutions.

The weaknesses of the design and evaluation procedures standard in medical informatics seem to be a close match to the strengths of ethnography. This suggests an interesting puzzle: why didn't researchers in this field invent ethnography, or some equivalent? Alternatively, why don't they engage social scientists to collect the sort of data that might help them to address the problem of user acceptance?

The answer to the first question is that they believe they did. In the expert systems world, the process known as knowledge acquisition, which involves debriefing experts and consulting written sources, is believed to provide accurate information about users, their problem-solving strategies, and the context of their work (ch. 3). The drawbacks of this approach (e.g., the predictable gaps between an expert's conscious models of reality and the complexity of real-life social processes) are simply not apparent from within the paradigm in which my informants work.

The answer to the second question again brings up the relationship between beliefs and perception. Early in my fieldwork among these scientists, I assumed that they were unaware of qualitative social science and that they would make use of ethnography (or collaborate with ethnographers) if only they knew of them. In time I realized that this inference was wrong. For well over a decade, a few researchers from anthropology and qualitative sociology have been working on the fringes of medical informatics, attempting to demonstrate that social science can help people in this field to meet their own goal of building computer systems that users will want to use (Cicourel 1990; Fafchamps 1991; Fafchamps, Young, and Tang 1991; Forsythe and Buchanan 1991; Forsythe, Buchanan, Osheroff, and Miller 1992; Kaplan 1987; Kaplan and Duchon 1988; Lundsgaarde, Fischer, and Steele 1981; Lundsgaarde 1987; Nyce and Graves 1990). In non-medical domains, Suchman and colleagues have been consistent advocates of the application of ethnographic techniques to system design (Suchman 1987; Greenbaum and Kyng 1991). Although this message has been published repeatedly in sources accessible to readers in medical informatics, the message itself has largely fallen on deaf ears. The ACMI statement mentioned above makes no mention of social science, treating the problem of user acceptance as a baffling phenomenon on which no real information exists. Standard operating procedures for problem definition, design, and evaluation have changed very little over time with respect to the issues raised in this paper. The values and assumptions that researchers in this field take for granted seem to make it very difficult for them to take seriously any approach that does not reflect their own formal, technical, quantitative biases.[8]

This situation is ironic. In attempting to explain why most medical expert systems sit unused on the shelf, people in the field speculate about external factors, with emphasis upon the cantankerous nature of users. As we have seen, however, much of the problem stems from their own understanding of science. The culture of medical informatics offers them procedures for problem formulation, design, system-building, and evaluation as well as a set of strong beliefs about the nature of science and scientific information. These beliefs are both partial and powerful; committed to them, the scientists cling to procedures that do not meet their own goals and fail to see a possible solution to the problem of user acceptance that arises from a source they do not value.

Finally, I want to consider power in a political sense. I have tried to explain from a conceptual standpoint why my informants carry on producing systems that the public doesn't use. As researchers, they are simply more interested in systems as technical objects than they are in assessing and meeting the needs of users. Thus, they overlook the question of users' needs while continuing to build systems that they find interesting and technically challenging. At the development end, most of these researchers are based in academic medicine. Although building medical expert systems might sound like a kind of service industry, academic computer specialists are under no real pressure from universities to produce products that medical consumers will want to use.

But what about the funding end? In the midst of a health care crisis in this country, with costs escalating and services declining, the government continues to pour millions of dollars into the development of systems that do not get used in medical care. Current system-building proposals tend to be justified in terms of concerns about health care delivery and to contain detailed sections on evaluation. Nevertheless, systems continue to be built that are not used in health care, and it is a rare evaluation that pays systematic attention to the question of a system's utility in a real-world work setting. How is this situation possible from a political standpoint? I believe that the answer lies in the nature of the field. Although medical informatics is growing rapidly, a small group of people continues to define the research issues and to sit on peer review panels. This "old boy network" (which includes a few women) is a small, homogeneous community. Individuals in charge of funding in Washington, D.C., belong to the same network as the senior scientists and clearly share the same research paradigm. For example, the past president of the main professional association in medical informatics is also the head of the major funding agency in this field. It is hardly surprising, then, that funders and senior researchers share the same agenda. What is missing from this agenda is the voice of users: potential users of medical expert systems are not part of the small, face-to-face community of decision-makers in this field, nor do they sit on review panels for proposals or journals. To borrow a term from Ardener, in medical informatics the voice of users is "muted" (Ardener 1975).

CONCLUSION

Cultural factors make a significant contribution to the problem of user acceptance of knowledge-based medical information systems. As we have seen, the scientists who build these systems tend to blame potential users for their failure to adopt this new technology on a widespread basis. However, observation suggests that an important source of the problem is to be found in the worldview of the scientists themselves: in the beliefs and assumptions that they bring to the system-building process and in the practice in which these values are expressed. Designed, built, and evaluated according to procedures that "delete the social" and mute the voice of users, most of these systems remain "on the shelf," a fact which is hardly surprising.

# CHAPTER TWO

# The Construction of Work in Artificial Intelligence

In contradistinction to the commonsense view of technology as value-free, and thus to be judged largely according to whether it "works" or not, a major theme of the developing anthropology of science and technology (Hess 1992) is that technological tools contain embedded values.[1] From an anthropological perspective, such tools embody values and assumptions held (often tacitly) by those who construct them. Thus, for example, tools of experimental high-energy physics embody beliefs about gender (Traweek 1988a); knowledge-based systems encode assumptions about the relation between plans and human action (Suchman 1987) and/or about the order of particular work processes (Sachs 1994; Suchman 1992); and a hypermedia system for high school students incorporates a cultural theory about choice, education, and the individualistic nature of human knowledge (Nyce and Bader 1993).

This implies that technology has a cultural dimension. As understood in interpretive anthropology, the approach taken in this paper, culture defines what people take for granted: the basic categories they use to make sense of the world and to decide how to act in it (Geertz 1973, 1983). In addition to the broader cultural background(s) in which any scientific practice takes place, academic disciplines define ways of viewing and acting in the world that can also be described as cultural. Thus, as scientists address the choices and problems that inevitably arise in the course of their practice (Pfaffenberger 1992: 498–9), the solutions they construct reflect the cultural realities of their own social and disciplinary milieux.

This paper takes a case from the expert systems community within artificial intelligence (AI) to examine how particular assumptions held by practitioners come to be embedded in the tools they construct. Expert systems are complex computer programs designed to do work that requires intelligent decision-making. As such, they embody explicit ideas about such matters as useful problem-solving strategies. Expert systems also embody some ideas that are less explicit, central among which are beliefs about the meaning of knowledge and work. In chapter 3, I address the *construction of knowledge* in AI, investigating what system-builders mean by "knowledge" and how their epistemological stance is incorporated in the expert systems they produce. Here I take up the related topic of the *construction of work* in AI. As with the construction of knowledge, the construction of work can be understood in two ways, both of which I propose to address. These are, first, the distinctive way in which the notion of work is understood by the practitioners to be described; and, second, the way in which this particular understanding of work affects their system-building procedures and thus the resultant systems. I will try to show (1) that practitioners apply the term "work" in a very selective manner to their own professional activities, and (2) that this selective approach carries over to the way in which they investigate the work of the human experts whose practice knowledge-based systems are intended to emulate. Then, I will suggest (3) that the resultant partial representation of expert knowledge encoded in the knowledge base of such systems affects the way the systems themselves finally work, contributing to their fallibility when encountering real-world situations.

The material presented here is part of an ongoing investigation of what one might call the "culture of artificial intelligence" (chs. 1, 3).[2] This research focuses on the relationship between the values and assumptions that a community of AI practitioners bring to their work, the practices that constitute that work, and the tools constructed in the course of that work. The AI specialists I describe view their professional work as science (and, in some cases, engineering), which they understand in positivist terms as being beyond or outside of culture. However, detailed observation of their daily work suggests that the truths and procedures of AI are in many ways culturally contingent. The scientists' work and the approach they take to it make sense in relation to a particular view of the world that is taken for granted in the laboratory. Documenting that worldview is a central goal of this research. However, what the scientists try to do doesn't always work as they believe it should, leading to confusions and ironies that I attempt to document as well.

Data for this research have been gathered in the course of an extended anthropological field study. Since 1986 I have been a full-time participant-observer in five different expert systems laboratories, four in academia and one in industry. The vast majority of that time has been spent in two of these labs. In order to help protect the identity of my informants, I will present the material below under the collective label "the Lab."

In addition to laboratory-based participant-observation, this research has involved taking part in meetings with representatives of various funding agencies, in national conferences, and in research and writing teams that have produced proposals and publications in AI and related fields. By moving in and out of a range of laboratory and other professional settings, I have attempted to study a scientific community rather than to focus exclusively upon the laboratories as bounded social entities. This community-centered approach to the study of science and technology follows that developed by Traweek (1988a), extending the laboratory-centered approach pioneered by Latour and Woolgar (1986), Knorr-Cetina (1981), and Lynch (1985).

BACKGROUND

## Expert Systems

Expert systems are constructed through a process known as "knowledge engineering" (ch. 3) by practitioners in AI. Some but not all of these practitioners identify themselves as "knowledge engineers." Each expert system is intended to automate decision-making processes normally undertaken by a human expert by capturing and coding in machine-readable form the background knowledge and rules of thumb ("heuristics") used by the expert to make decisions in a particular subject area ("domain"). This information is encoded in the system's "knowledge base," which is then manipulated by the system's "inference engine" in order to reach conclusions relating to the tasks at hand.[3]

Building an expert system typically involves carrying out the following steps:

1. Collecting information from one or more human informants and/or from documentary sources.

2. Ordering that information into procedures (e.g., rules and constraints) relevant to the operations that the prospective system is intended to perform.

3. Designing or adapting a computer program to apply these rules and constraints in performing the designated operations.

The first two steps in this series—that is, the gathering of information and its translation into machine-readable form—comprise the process known as "knowledge acquisition." The early stages of knowledge acquisition often include extended face-to-face interviewing of one or more experts, a process sometimes referred to as "knowledge elicitation."

## Falling Off the Knowledge Cliff

Knowledge-based systems contain stored information (referred to as "knowledge") plus encoded procedures for manipulating that knowledge. One problem with such systems to date is that they are both narrow and brittle. That is, while they may function satisfactorily within narrow limits—a specific application, problem area, or domain—they tend to fail rapidly and completely when moved very far from those limits or when faced with situations that the system-builders did n )t anticipate. This is referred to as the tendency of such systems to "fall off the knowledge cliff."[4] Various knowledge-related problems can befall systems in the real world. I will provide two examples that relate to the theme of this paper; in different ways, each reflects the problem of tacit knowledge. A well-known example of a knowledge-related failure is provided by MYCIN, one of the first expert systems for medical diagnosis. Given a male patient with a bacterial infection, MYCIN suggested that one likely source of infection might be a prior amniocentesis. While this is absurd, no one had thought to build into the system's knowledge base the information that men don't get pregnant. Therefore, it did not prune "amniocentesis" from the menu of possible sources of infection in men (Buchanan and Shortliffe 1984: 692). Information about where babies come from is representative of a large class of knowledge that experts might not think to explain to interviewers, but which is clearly essential for correct inference in certain areas of human activity. Without such taken-for-granted background knowledge about the world, expert systems tend to fall off the knowledge cliff. In the case of MYCIN, information was *omitted* from a knowledge base, presumably because of the system-builders' tacit assumption that everybody knows that men don't get pregnant. This cultural assumption works well in the context of communication between humans over the age of six, but is inappropriate when applied to computers.

In a case documented by Sachs (1994), on the other hand, a knowledge-related problem arose because inappropriate information was *built into* a knowledge base. Sachs describes an expert system for inventory control that cannot accommodate the information that the actual supply of a given part differs from what the system "believes" it should be according to assumptions encoded by the system-builders. She reports that seasoned users sometimes resort to "tricking" the system, knowingly entering false information in order to work around these built-in assumptions.[5] We may assume that people on the shop floor are perfectly aware that work doesn't always take place according to official procedures. However, it appears that this piece of background knowledge may not have been built into the knowledge base in such a way as to accommodate the complexity of real-life situations. The result is a system that falls off the knowledge cliff, able to function as it should only if users sometimes distort their input to conform to the internal "reality" encoded in the system.

Within AI, problems like this have been attributed to three causes. First, the limits of technology: at present it isn't feasible to store enough "knowledge" to enable expert systems to be broadly applicable. Second, such systems don't themselves contain so-called "deep models" of the problem areas within which they work, either because there is no adequate theory in that area or because the technology for representing models is not adequate (Karp and Wilkins 1989). And third, expert systems don't have what AI people refer to as "common sense" (Lenat and Feigenbaum 1987; McCarthy 1984).

Research in AI is attempting to solve these problems. For example, there is now a massive effort under way to try to embed common sense into expert systems. One such effort is the CYC project at Microelectronics and Computer Technology Corporation (MCC) in Texas (Guha and Lenat 1990; Lenat and Guha 1990; Lenat, Prakash, and Shepherd 1986); CYC is an enormous computerized knowledge base intended to encode the knowledge necessary to read and understand "any encyclopedia article" (Guha and Lenat 1990: 34). In the words of its builders, "To build CYC, we must encode all the world's knowledge down to some level of detail; there is no way to finesse this" (Lenat, Prakash, and Shepherd 1986: 75). The intended outcome of this project will be a generalized commonsense knowledge base that will apply to a wide range of systems and thus keep those systems from falling off the knowledge cliff.

As a participant-observer in the world of expert systems, I have a somewhat different perspective than AI specialists on why these systems are narrow and brittle. Current technical and representational capabilities may well impose limitations, as my informants insist; I am not in a position to evaluate that claim. After observing the process of building the systems, however, I believe that there is another source of difficulty that also affects the way expert systems perform but of which there is very little discussion in AI. In my view, some of the problems that the scientists attribute to the limitations of technology are actually reflections of implicit assumptions and conceptual orientations of the system-builders themselves.

In other publications I have pursued this theme with respect to the meaning and implications for design of three basic concepts in AI: the notions of knowledge (ch. 3), information (Forsythe, Buchanan, Osheroff, and Miller 1992), and evaluation (Forsythe and Buchanan 1991).[6] All of these concepts are interpreted more formally and narrowly in AI than they are in, say, anthropology. The different assumptions about the nature of knowledge held by AI specialists and anthropologists are illustrated by their different reactions to the CYC project mentioned above. To many researchers in AI, this project makes obvious sense. Since they tend to see knowledge as "out there" and as universal in nature, building a generalized commonsense knowledge base seems to them a challenging but meaningful and worthwhile goal. In contrast, anthropologists typically react to this idea as absurd; given the anthropological view of commonsense (and other) knowledge as *cultural* and therefore local in nature (Geertz 1983: ch. 4), the notion of universally applicable common sense is an oxymoron. Thus, if we regard academic disciplines as "intellectual villages," as Geertz suggests (Geertz 1983: 157), the villagers of AI and cultural anthropology see the world in distinctly different ways.

## WHAT IS THE WORK OF ARTIFICIAL INTELLIGENCE?

Continuing this exploration into the shared assumptions and practices of the world of AI, I turn now to the way in which system-builders construct the notion of work. Understanding how they view work (their own as well as that of the experts whose work their systems are designed to emulate or replace) illuminates a good deal about why expert systems are narrow and brittle—and thus at risk of falling off the knowledge cliff. Beginning with a brief description of the work setting, I will present some material on the way in which Lab members describe their own work and then contrast that with what I actually see them doing in the Lab.

The Lab consists of a series of largely open-plan rooms with desks and carrels for graduate students and visiting researchers. Individual offices are provided for the Lab head, members of the research staff, and senior secretarial and administrative personnel, and there is a seminar room that doubles as a library. Most work rooms contain whiteboards, typically covered with lists and diagrams written in ink of various colors; and nearly every desk, carrel, and office is equipped with a terminal or networked personal computer linked to one of the Lab's four laser printers.

All Lab members do some of their work on these computers, work which is in a sense invisible to the observer. This presents something of a problem for the fieldworker wishing to record details of their practice. Walking through the research areas, what one sees are individuals (mostly male) seated in swivel chairs in front of large computer screens, sometimes typing and sometimes staring silently at the screen. Occasionally two or three individuals gather in front of a screen to confer over a problem. The products of this labor are also largely invisible, since the systems themselves are stored in the computers. They manifest themselves in the form of diagrams or segments of code that appear in windows on the computer screens and are sometimes transferred to "hard copy" (that is, printed out on paper).

Wondering what it means to "do AI," I have asked many practitioners to describe their own work. Their answers invariably focus on one or more of the following: problem-solving, writing code, and building systems. These three tasks are seen as aspects of a single process: one writes code (that is, programs a computer) in the course of building a system, which in turn is seen as a means of discovering the solution to a problem. The central work of AI, then, is problem-solving; writing code and building systems are strategies for accomplishing that work. One scientist said:

> Every first version (of a system) ought to be a throwaway. You can work on conceptualizing the problem through the programming. . . . Generally speaking we don't know how to solve the problem when it's handed to us. It's handed over to us when there's no mathematical solution. . . . You start solving the problem by beginning to program, and then the computer becomes your ally in the process instead of your enemy.

This view of AI is presented consistently, not only in talking to me but also in spontaneous conversations in the Lab, in textbooks, and in lectures to graduate students.

However, we get a somewhat different picture of the work of AI if we take an observational approach to this question, looking at what the scientists in the Lab actually spend their days doing. Lab members perform a wide range of tasks, some carried out individually and some collectively. They do write code, build systems, and solve problems. But they also do a large number of other things in the course of their work day. These tasks—many of which are not mentioned when Lab members characterize their work—include the following.

First, there are meetings. Lab members spend an enormous amount of time every week in face-to-face meetings, of which there are many sorts.

1. Lab meetings: There are regular meetings for the purpose of Lab management and for keeping up with who is doing what. These are of two sorts. First, there is a general meeting attended by the Lab head, staff researchers, and graduate students. At this meeting everyone reports on what has been accomplished during the previous week and what is planned the coming week. Second, there is a periodic meeting of what is known as the "Lab exec," which is attended by the Lab head, the staff researchers, and senior secretarial and administrative staff. At this meeting, discussions take place concerning issues of policy.

2. Project meetings: Roughly half a dozen major research projects are based in the Lab, all of which involve collaboration between Lab members and researchers from other departments within (and in some cases outside) the university. These projects meet on a regular basis in the Lab seminar room, some weekly and some less often.

3. Research seminars: Several research seminars are run from the Lab on themes central to the Lab's research agenda.

4. Formal meetings of committees and groups outside the Lab: departmental faculty meetings, interdisciplinary program meetings, meetings with division units, meetings with the Dean, etc.

5. Informal meetings with colleagues from the department, from other departments, from elsewhere in the university, and from other universities for such purposes as project development, keeping abreast of events, formulating political strategy, attempting to mediate disputes, etc.

6. Meetings with current, former, and potential students for the purpose of guidance and recruiting.

7. Meetings in connection with work for outside institutions: These include review boards of professional societies, editorial boards, academic institutions, and funding agencies, management and program committees of professional societies, and so forth.

8. Reviewing for journals, conferences, and funding agencies.

9. Conferences, academic meetings.

In addition to all these face-to-face meetings, Lab members carry out a wide variety of other tasks, including the following:

10. Communication with colleagues, students, and others that is not face-to-face: This includes communication by letter and telephone, but consists increasingly of communication by means of electronic mail (e-mail). All Lab members have e-mail accounts through which they can communicate equally easily with people in the next office and with people in other countries. This communication is free to Lab members, and they spend a good deal of time at it. The head of the Lab estimates that he spends 20 percent of his time on e-mail.

11. Seeking funding: The laboratory runs on soft money. Only the head of the Lab receives a full-time academic salary, and even he is responsible for raising his own summer salary in grant money. Money for part of the secretarial and administrative salaries and for the research scientists' and graduate students' salaries must be raised through grants. Thus, a good deal of laboratory work time is spent in investigating sources of money, in project development, in proposal writing and editing, in budgeting proposed projects, and in politicking in support of these proposals. The head of the Lab estimates that he spends at least 20 percent of his time in pursuit of funding.

12. Teaching courses: This includes lecture time and course preparation time (for teaching staff).

13. Taking courses: This includes lecture time and studying time (for graduate students).

14. Writing papers, editing, and preparing outside lectures.

15. Lab and departmental administration, including budgeting.

16. Clerical and administrative work: The Lab secretaries and administrators do this full-time, with occasional help from work-study students and from other secretaries in the department. In addition, Lab members do a good deal of photocopying for themselves.

17. Hardware and software maintenance and upgrading: This includes virus checking, installing new versions of operating systems and applications software on the dozen or so computers in the Lab, maintaining software compatibility, etc.

18. Personal file and directory maintenance on the computer: The computer analog of housekeeping.

19. And, finally, Lab members write code, build systems, and solve problems.

Few of these tasks will be surprising to academic readers; after all, this is a composite of a university research laboratory. There are, however, some interesting things about this list when viewed in relation to what practitioners *say* about what their work consists of. To begin with, there is a striking disparity between the self-description and the observational data on what these scientists do at work. Two points stand out here. First, the tasks that Lab members can be seen to do on a regular basis are far more various than their own description suggests: that self-description is highly selective. Even if we look only at the realm of activity concerned with computers, their self-description is selective. Computers require backup, maintenance, and repair; software requires updating; compatibility must be maintained; and virus-checkers must be kept up-to-date. But although all Lab members engage in these tasks, no informant has ever mentioned them as part of the work of AI.

Second, not only is the scientists' description of their work selective, since no Lab members spend all of their time writing code and building systems, but in at least one case it is totally false. The head of the Lab does no such work at all: his time is fully taken up with laboratory management, fundraising, and teaching. As the following dialogue illustrates, however, he is apologetic about the fact that he doesn't actually do such work.

*Scientist:*       You're getting a skewed view of AI when you look at what I do. I'm not writing any code!

*Anthropologist:*   When was the last time you wrote some code?

*Scientist:*       Seriously, you mean, as opposed to just playing around? Eighty or '81, I suppose, for [company name], when I was doing some consulting for them.

*Anthropologist:*   So are you doing AI when I observe you?

*Scientist:*       Well, when I'm working with [students], I think, yes. Because that involves conceptualizing, defining problems, and that's an important part of AI. But I have to leave it up to them to write the code.

This senior scientist concedes that he has not worked on code for system-building for over ten years. Yet he, too, clearly shares the belief that writing code and building systems are what constitute the "real work" of AI.

In describing their work as writing code and building systems, practitioners are not being absent-minded. They are perfectly aware that their day includes many other pursuits besides writing code; however, they are reluctant to label these other pursuits as "work." When I pursued this question with several informants, they all made some kind of distinction among their daily pursuits. One distinguished between "real work" and "other stuff he had to do"; another made a distinction between "work" and "pseudo-work." "Real work" or "real AI" turns out to involve conceptualization and problem-solving, writing code, and building systems; "pseudo-work" or "other stuff," on the other hand, includes most other tasks, such as attending meetings, doing e-mail, recruiting faculty, looking for research funding, and writing recommendations. When asked what their work entailed, then, these scientists described only the "real work," not the "pseudo-work" on which they also spend a great deal of their time.

Some examples will help to clarify the boundary between "real work" and "pseudo-work." First, not all kinds of computer use count as real work: recall that reading and sending e-mail was labeled "pseudo-work." Second, not all kinds of programming count as work, as is illustrated by the following interchange between two students.

*Anthropologist* (to student 1, sitting at a terminal):    What are you doing?
*Student 1*:    Working on a spreadsheet program, actually.
*Student 2* (interjects from neighboring desk):    Using, not working on.
*Student 1*:    Using it.

My informants distinguish between using or working *with* a piece of software, and working *on* it. Student 1 was working with the spreadsheet as a user, but was not changing the code that defines the underlying spreadsheet platform. The students agreed that this operation should be called "using the program," not working on it. Since using a spreadsheet generally involves doing some programming to customize it to one's purposes, this is not a distinction between programming and not programming. Rather, it refers to what is being programmed. They apply the term "working on" to programming that modifies the basic code. What they are doing, then, is restricting their use of "work" to what they think of as "real AI": building systems.

Third, other aspects of the boundary between work and pseudo-work are evident in the distinction Lab members make between "doing" and "talking." Work is doing things, not talking about doing them; talking about things is not doing work. This distinction was illustrated during a talk with the Lab head about a large interdisciplinary project based in the Lab. When I expressed concern that project members seemed to have committed themselves to a conceptual position that might turn out to be counterproductive in the long run, the Lab head replied in astonishment, "But we haven't done any work yet!" At this point, members working on the project in question had been meeting regularly for about a year. From an anthropological point of view, a great deal of work had already been done by project members, including reading, discussing, writing two major proposals, carrying out preliminary fieldwork in two medical clinics, and beginning the process of formal knowledge elicitation for a medical expert system. What no one had yet done, however, was to *write code* for the prospective system. Since to AI specialists the central meaning of "work" is writing code and building systems, no real work had yet taken place on that project.

Lab members clearly categorize activities differently from anthropologists, for whom developing a common conceptual approach to a research project (thinking and talking about doing) would certainly count as real work. Since the Lab members see themselves as paid to build systems, general discussions of epistemological issues that do not relate to specific systems under construction are seen as a waste of time. Such discussions might well be fun (one informant characterized them as "play"), but they do not count as work:

> If my work is to build systems, and I'm talking about epistemological issues, there would be a question in my mind about whether I was doing my work or wasting time. . . . [There] might be some guilt there.

Discussing the topic of this paper, a Lab member grinned and explained his own philosophy (partly in jest) as, "Just shut your mouth and do the work!" He wrote these words on the nearest whiteboard. Knowing that I had been learning LISP, the computer language in which Lab members build their systems, he then playfully translated the message into LISP code: (AND [shut mouth] [do work]).

What should we understand by the selectivity in the scientists' use of the term "work" in describing their daily activities in the Lab? What is the significance of their consistent division of these activities into legitimate and illegitimate forms of work? I suggest that this selectivity is meaningful and that it conveys some important things about Lab members' implicit assumptions.

First, the way in which they construct their work reveals their thoroughgoing technical orientation, which I refer to elsewhere as their "engineering ethos" (ch. 3). In describing their work as problem-solving, Lab members could be referring to many of the things they regularly do in the Lab; the list given above includes numerous tasks that could be described as "problem-solving." However, what they actually mean by that term is formal or *technical* problem-solving. This does *not* include resolving social, political, or interactional problems, although these too arise in the course of their workday. Thus, the "problem-solving" which these scientists define as their work is formal, bounded, and very narrowly defined. Problem-solving in this sense is what you do while sitting alone for hours at the computer. In adopting this description of their own work, the scientists are deleting the social, to use Leigh Star's evocative phrase (Star 1991). This can be seen in two senses. The focus on writing code and building systems leaves out the fact that a significant proportion of their daily professional activities is actually social in nature—recall all those meetings and seminars. Furthermore, even writing code and building systems takes place in a social and institutional context, necessitating interaction with fellow project members, experts, funders, and so on. Thus, the scientists' description of their own work is highly decontextualized.

This selective description reflects an idealized representation of their work. The practitioners are describing what they see as the essence of their work, which is also the part they most enjoy doing. Their construction of their work thus focuses not on what they actually do all of the time, but rather on what they would *like* to spend all their time doing if only the unpleasant demands of everyday life took care of themselves. From an anthropological standpoint, these scientists seem strikingly casual about the distinction between the ideal and the real. Asked a question about what their work entails, Lab members consistently respond with an answer that seems far more ideal than real.

I suggest that the selectivity of their description of their own work has symbolic meaning. The particular activities the scientists list as "real work" are those in terms of which they construct their own identity as "real AI" scientists. In the Lab, possession of these skills is used on occasion as a boundary marker to distinguish between those who belong in an AI lab and those who do not. For example, one day at a Lab meeting, a practitioner opposed a suggestion of mine with the comment, "Anyone who can't program Unix or figure out what's wrong with a Mac shouldn't be in this lab." Now the fact is that there is an enormous overlap between what this researcher does all day in the Lab and what I do there as a participant-observer: we attend many of the same meetings, read some of the same literature, write papers, seek funding (from some of the same agencies), talk with many of the same students and colleagues, and spend hours every day sitting at the same type of computer. In fact, just about the *only* activities we do not share are writing code and building systems. Since these are the activities that define "real AI," however, they can also be used to define a boundary between those who belong in the Lab and those who do not.[7] My point is not to object to such boundary-drawing, but rather to demonstrate the fact that the professional activities that take place in the Lab have differential symbolic weight.

To sum up my argument thus far, practitioners can be observed to perform a wide range of tasks during the work day. But when asked what their work consists of, they consistently mention only a few of these tasks. "Work" as my informants construct it is not about interpersonal communication or most of the other daily activities one can observe in the Lab, although all Lab members spend a large proportion of their time on these activities. Instead, work is about finding solutions to formal problems through the process of building systems. Work is thus defined in terms of isolated task-performance that involves solving logical problems, but not interpersonal ones. This is why laboratory management doesn't strike the head of the Lab as "real work."

DISCUSSION

The starting point of this investigation was the apparently simple question, "What is the work of AI?" Complexity arose as it became clear that practitioners describe their work in a way that leaves out a great deal. These scientists represent their work in terms of an ideal model that seems to have symbolic meaning to them but that in its focus on formal problem-solving is at best a partial representation of what their daily practice actually entails.

The long list of activities left out of this description (see above) may be familiar to the academic reader, who may also resent administrative and other duties of the sort that AI practitioners perform but do not consider to be "real work." However, we should not allow familiarity to blind us to the significance of the considerable discrepancy between the scientists' representation of their work and their observable practice. By systematically discounting a substantial proportion of their work, they are engaging in large-scale deletion (Star 1991: 266–7). Much of what they actually do in the Lab is thereby rendered invisible, relegated to a category of unimportant or illegitimate work. Among these deleted activities are the many acts of social, intellectual, and material maintenance that lie outside the realm of formal problem-solving. This systematic deletion is taken for granted in the world of expert systems: in anthropological terms, it is part of the local culture.

The selectivity with which system-builders represent their own work is interesting from a number of standpoints. This discussion will focus on two of them. They are first, the implications of the practitioners' concept of work for the way they go about knowledge acquisition; and second, what this may imply in turn for the way expert systems function in the real world.

## Implications for Knowledge Acquisition

When carrying out knowledge elicitation to gather material for the knowledge base of an expert system, my informants approach the experts' work with the same selectivity that they bring to characterizing their own work. The scientists' construction of their experts' work is also partial, idealized, formal, and decontextualized; it is characterized by the same deletions outlined above.[8]

In describing their own work, the scientists conflate the ideal and the real, making little distinction between observable practice and verbal descriptions of that practice. Their approach to knowledge elicitation reflects the same way of thinking. The purpose of an expert system is to perform the work of a given human expert; the knowledge encoded in the system is intended to reflect what that expert actually does. However, knowledge engineering rarely involves observing experts at work. Instead, what practitioners do is to interview them—that is, they collect experts' reports of what they do at work, apparently failing to take into account that (as we have seen in the case of the system-builders themselves) people's descriptions of their own work processes can be highly selective.[9] In actuality, the information recorded during knowledge elicitation is even more distanced than this from observable practice: what goes into the knowledge base of an expert system is in fact the knowledge engineer's model of the expert's model of his or her own work.

In response to this argument, practitioners tend to reply that they *do* watch the expert at work. However, what they mean by this again reflects the selective view of work that I am attempting to describe. Experts are indeed often asked to do "work" for the purpose of knowledge engineering; however, this usually does not mean demonstrating their normal work patterns in their customary occupational setting. Instead, what they are asked to do is to perform isolated tasks or to solve formal problems that are taken to represent that work. The experts' verbal commentary as they solve such problems is taken as data on their work performance in its normal setting. For example, for a system designed to do medical diagnosis, system-builders asked doctors to read case histories and give a verbal account of how they would diagnose them; for a system designed to diagnose automotive problems, a mechanic was asked how he went about deciding what was wrong with a car; for a system to simulate student reasoning in physics, students of varying degrees of expertise were given problems to solve from an undergraduate textbook. As representations of actual work in the world, these contrived tasks are partial in precisely the same way as the scientists' representations of their own work. Since such tasks are narrow and formal—"paper puzzles" as opposed to genuine problems encountered in a real world context—they leave out a great deal of the normal work process. In addition, since it is customary in knowledge engineering to work with only one expert per system (the physics project designated the best student problem-solver as the expert), conventional elicitation procedures are likely to overlook variations in the way different skillful individuals approach the same task.

Some practitioners are aware that there are drawbacks in these conventional procedures. For example, a textbook describes the limitations of relying upon experts' descriptions of their rules and heuristics for solving a problem. The authors attempt to overcome some of these limitations by suggesting that the work of repairing toasters be analyzed by having "Frank Fixit" bring a toaster to the knowledge elicitation session in order to demonstrate his diagnostic skills (Scott, Clayton, and Gibson 1991). But even where the object "diagnosed" is actually used in the knowledge acquisition process, the work tends to be observed and analyzed out of context. The anthropological emphasis upon *situated* understanding (Suchman 1987) stresses the importance of seeing how people approach problems in the settings in which they are accustomed to work. This is not usually done, however: expert systems are still built without the system-builder(s) ever visiting the expert's place of work.

Approaching knowledge elicitation as they do, practitioners learn little about the informal social and institutional processes that are an essential part of work in real-life settings. For example, faced with a problematic diagnosis, physicians often call a colleague (Weinberg, Ullian, Richards, and Cooper 1981); if official rules and procedures do not suit the needs of a particular patient or situation, they figure out how to get around those rules.[10]

In relying on interviews plus data on problem-solving in contrived situations, system-builders acquire a decontextualized picture of the expert's work. As in their representation of their own work, they discount much of what experts actually do.

To sum up, the "knowledge" that the scientists put into their knowledge bases is narrow: it simply leaves out a lot. The models of behavior it includes are encoded without much information on either the contexts in terms of which these models have meaning or on how the models are actually translated into action in real-life situations. In that sense, this knowledge is brittle as well. In short, standard knowledge elicitation procedures reflect—and replicate—the same deletions that practitioners apply to their own work.

## Implications for Expert Systems

I have argued that there is a parallel between the way my informants construct their own work and the way they construct their experts' work in the course of knowledge elicitation. In both cases we see the influence of a formal and decontextualized notion of work. The final step of my argument is to draw the conclusion that this formal and decontextualized notion of work contributes to the construction of expert systems that are narrow and brittle—and thus vulnerable to failure when faced with the complexity of work processes in the real world. The system described by Sachs (1994) and discussed above fell off the knowledge cliff at least in part because it incorporated a normative model of the work processes that it was designed to monitor. This idealized representation was apparently too partial and inflexible to function as intended in the real world. I suggest that the scientists who built this system may unintentionally have contributed to its fragility by assuming that actual work processes and contexts would conform to the idealized representations of them presumably offered by their expert(s). This expectation, which reflects the culture of AI, confuses the ideal and the real. In contrast, perhaps because of their fieldwork experience, anthropologists tend to make the opposite assumption. If anything, they assume that normative rules and everyday action are not related in a simple way (ch. 3; Geertz 1973, 1983). I assume that the builders of this system followed the conventional knowledge elicitation procedures described above and did not systematically observe the workplace(s) in which their system was to be fielded. Had they done so, they would surely have discovered that problem-solving in real-world contexts does not (and indeed cannot) always conform to the simplified "typical" cases offered by experts. Perhaps the system could then have been designed to "expect" deviations from the ideal.

In summary, the characteristic deletions in the scientists' representation of their own work are replicated not only in their system-building procedures, but also in the technology itself. I suggest that if today's expert systems tend to fall off the knowledge cliff, one cause may be the shallowness of the information encoded in those systems on the nature of expert work and the nature of the knowledge that experts bring to such work (ch. 3).

CONCLUSION

The case presented in this paper supports the growing body of evidence from the anthropology of science and technology that knowledge-based systems are far from value-free (Sachs 1994; Suchman 1987, 1992). Elsewhere I have tried to show that such systems incorporate tacit assumptions about the nature of knowledge (ch. 3); here I contend that they also embody assumptions about the nature of work.

There is a striking symmetry between what the practitioners seem to assume about the world and the characteristics of the systems they build to operate in the world. They do not seem aware of this symmetry, however. Given that fundamental assumptions about the nature of knowledge and work are simply taken for granted, the process by which system-builders embed these beliefs in the tools they build is unlikely to reflect intentionality. Rather, as choices arise in the system-building process, tacit beliefs influence decision-making by default, in a way that anthropologists describe as cultural. Intentional or not, some of the practitioners' fundamental beliefs are replicated in the system-building process, with significant implications for the resulting technology.

The scientists I have described are unlikely to agree with this point of view: as we have seen, they tend to blame the inflexibility of expert systems on the limitations of current technology and representational capabilities. But the connection I have tried to delineate has nothing to do with the limitations of technology. Rather, it concerns one of the non-technical factors that practitioners often discount (Forsythe and Buchanan 1992): their own tacit assumptions, which among other things help to shape their knowledge acquisition procedures. If they understand "real work" to mean only formal, technical, decontextualized problem-solving, and if their information-gathering procedures reflect that perception, then it is hardly surprising that the expert systems they produce are narrow and brittle. Ironically, through their own default assumptions, these scientists may be helping to push their own systems off the knowledge cliff.

# CHAPTER THREE

# Engineering Knowledge: The Construction of Knowledge in Artificial Intelligence

For social scientists interested in the nature of knowledge, the idea of artificial intelligence (AI) is fascinating and provocative. AI research raises fundamental questions concerning culture, cognition, knowledge, and power as well as central philosophical and methodological problems.[1] Visionaries in the AI community believe that computers will increasingly be able to duplicate human expertise (e.g., Feigenbaum and McCorduck 1984; Feigenbaum, McCorduck, and Nii, 1988). Skeptics reply that because of the nature of knowledge, machines can support human expertise but not completely replace it.[2] This debate reflects very different assumptions about what knowledge is, how it is produced, and what would be required to automate the manipulation of knowledge in a meaningful way.

This paper explores the construction of knowledge in AI. By this I mean first, the way in which the concept of knowledge is understood by a particular group of scientists; and second, the way in which they go about producing knowledge as they understand the concept. I will argue that the scientists to be described share a distinctly restricted notion of what "knowledge" means and that this notion has important implications for their understanding of what their work entails, for the way in which they do that work, and for the products of that work. Known as knowledge engineers, my informants are members of the expert systems community within AI. The tools they design and construct are the complex computer programs known as knowledge-based or expert systems.[3]

The approach I will take is that of interpretive cultural anthropology, grounding the analysis in the attempt to understand what events mean to the people involved (Geertz 1973, 1983). Anthropologists typically pursue such understanding by undertaking long-term field research using the ethnographic method of participant observation (Ellen 1984; Werner and Schoepfle

1987). The anthropological tradition of extended field research stems in part from the recognition that in human affairs, the relation between beliefs and practice is invariably complex. In any given situation, what people believe that they should do, what they report that they do, and what they can be seen to do by an outside observer may all differ somewhat.[4] However, in the absence of systematic participant observation, such disparities are difficult to detect. If we base our study of science solely on scientists' self-reports, we may fail to realize what the reported actions or tools actually consist of; if we look only at observed practice, we may miss what particular objects or actions mean to the scientists involved; and if we limit ourselves to introspection about a particular problem addressed by scientists, we may learn little or nothing about how the scientists themselves approach the problem.

In order to understand how the "engineering" of knowledge is understood within the field of AI, therefore, I embarked upon an extended field study. Since 1986 I have been a full-time participant-observer in five different expert systems laboratories in the United States, four in academia and one in industry. Most of my time has been divided between two of these labs, the second of which was created when a senior member of the first left to start a new laboratory. Since there is a good deal in common between these two labs, and in order to help protect the identity of my informants, I present data from both under the collective label "the Lab."

In addition to laboratory-based participant-observation, I have in connection with this research taken part in numerous meetings with representatives of funding agencies, in national conferences, and in research and writing teams that have produced proposals and publications in AI and related fields. By moving in and out of a range of laboratory and other professional settings, I have attempted to study a scientific community rather than to focus exclusively upon the laboratories as bounded social entities. This community-centered approach to the study of science and technology follows that developed by Traweek (1988a), extending the laboratory-centered approach pioneered by such researchers as Latour and Woolgar (1986), Knorr-Cetina (1981), and Lynch (1985).

Initially, my research focused on the methods by which expert systems are constructed. Talking with AI professionals, I had been struck by the apparent parallels between the process that they call "knowledge acquisition" (see below) and what anthropologists do in the course of field research.[5] However, these seemingly parallel endeavors were clearly thought of quite differently in the two disciplines. Whereas anthropologists devote considerable energy to pondering methodological, ethical, and philosophical aspects of field research,[6] knowledge acquisition seemed to be undertaken in a rather unexamined way. Asked how they went about the task of gathering knowledge for their expert systems, the knowledge engineers I met tended to look surprised and say, "We just do it." Piqued by this straightforward approach to a task that anthropologists view as complex, I decided to investigate the ways in which knowledge engineers conceptualize and carry out the process of knowledge acquisition. As the fieldwork progressed, consideration of the values and assumptions that lead knowledge engineers to approach knowledge acquisition as they do raised my interest in broader questions. The research became an ongoing investigation of the relationship among the beliefs that a community of scientists bring to their work, the practice that constitutes that work, and the characteristics of the tools they construct in the course of that work.[7]

Such an investigation is a highly reflexive enterprise. As an anthropologist studying a scientific community engaged in formulating knowledge descriptions, I found myself faced with the necessity of formulating a knowledge description. Describing the epistemological stance of my informants inevitably reveals my own as well. Implicit in the ethnographic description below, the contrast in our perspectives is made explicit in the discussion that follows. This paper thus constitutes a kind of dialogue between contrasting voices—theirs and mine, observed and observer—about the nature of knowledge.

Finally, the paper is a critique of some aspects of AI. Drawing upon my ethnographic material, I raise questions about the conception of knowledge taken for granted by my informants as well as the procedures they use to "acquire" knowledge for the purpose of building expert systems. I suggest that the knowledge engineers' assumptions have some unintended negative consequences for their own practice, for the systems they build, and thus (potentially at least) for the broader society. By drawing attention to the impact of scientists' values upon scientific practice and its outcomes, I hope to encourage careful reflection on the part of practitioners of AI as well as a degree of caution among members of the public and scholars of other disciplines who may look to AI for guidance.

## Artificial Intelligence and the Social Study of Science[8]

Artificial intelligence has been the topic of a good deal of debate recently in this journal (*Social Studies of Science*).[9] Much of the discussion has focused upon the attempt to "prove" or "refute" the strong program by establishing whether or not machine discovery is possible and—more broadly—upon the question of whether or not AI has achieved or can ever achieve its "goals" or its "promise." Two aspects of this debate stand out from an anthropological viewpoint. First, the analysis to date has been largely acultural; that is, it attempts to address questions of (purported) truth or falsity rather than questions of meaning.[10] Second, claims and counter-claims in this debate have been put forward with little reference to data either on what AI practitioners actually do (as opposed to what they hope or claim to do), or on what they mean by the words they use to describe their goals and accomplishments.[11] The resultant exchanges reveal much about the divergent perspectives of the parties involved, but less about the practice of AI.

This paper differs both in taking a cultural approach and in focusing upon what AI specialists actually do in the laboratory. Information of this sort is necessary to understand both what these scientists are attempting to achieve and the attitudes and assumptions that inform their work. After all, what AI practitioners mean by the words they use is not always what commentators from other disciplines take them to mean. Much of the debate about whether intelligence has been or ever could be automated turns upon the different worldviews that various parties bring to the argument. Largely tacit, such differences affect individual perspectives in a way that anthropologists understand as cultural.

## Expert Systems and Knowledge Acquisition

Expert systems are designed to emulate human expertise; they are constructed using computer languages that can represent and manipulate symbolic information. Each system is intended to automate decision-making processes normally undertaken by a given human "expert" by capturing and coding in machine-readable form the background knowledge and rules of thumb ("heuristics") used by the expert to make decisions in a particular subject area ("domain"). This information is encoded in the system's "knowledge base," which is then manipulated by the system's "inference engine" in order to reach conclusions relating to the tasks at hand. To date, expert systems have been developed that perform such tasks as making medical diagnoses (MYCIN, developed at Stanford; QMR, developed at the University of Pittsburgh), predicting the location of mineral deposits (Prospector, developed at SRI), and aiding the process of drilling for oil (Dipmeter Advisor, developed at Schlumberger).[12]

Building an expert system typically involves the following steps:

1. Collecting information from one or more human informants and/or from documentary sources.

2. Ordering that information into procedures (e.g., rules and constraints) relevant to the operations that the prospective system is intended to perform.

3. Designing or adapting a computer program to apply these rules and constraints in performing the designated operations.

The first two steps in this series—that is, the gathering of information and its translation into machine-readable form—comprise the process known as "knowledge acquisition." Knowledge engineers are regarded as specialists in this task. The early stages of knowledge acquisition often include extended face-to-face interviewing of one or more experts by the knowledge engineer(s). This interview process will be referred to as "knowledge elicitation."

## Knowledge Elicitation

Knowledge engineers distinguish between "expertise" and "common sense." Expertise is seen as a particular way of thinking that is possessed by a certain category of human beings labeled "experts."

> Experts have rich structures and reasoning abilities. . . . Experts have stored rich representations of facts, objects and their attributes, as well as a set of inference rules that connect constellations of facts for use in problem-solving situations (Olson and Rueter 1987: 153, 166).

People perceived as experts tend to be highly paid and very senior in their particular occupational hierarchy. The purpose of knowledge elicitation is to collect such an individual's expertise in order (as one informant said) to "clone him."

Knowledge elicitation at the Lab involves face-to-face interviews which last about one to two hours, occur roughly once or twice a fortnight, and extend over a period of months or years. These interviews most often involve one knowledge engineer and one expert. However, some projects use teams of knowledge engineers, experts, or both.

Before meeting with their expert, knowledge engineers attempt to learn something about the problem domain by reading textbooks and other literature where available. Knowledge elicitation is seen as a means of filling in gaps in this written material. Since "expertise" to them means mainly textbook knowledge (as opposed to "common sense"), the Lab's knowledge engineers prefer domains for which written material does exist. In practice, this means that most of the expert systems they produce pertain to academic and scientific fields such as medicine, chemistry, physics, and engineering. The advantage of such domains from the knowledge engineers' standpoint is that they are highly codified, which reduces the amount of knowledge elicitation seen as necessary. This is particularly true of medical diagnosis, probably the Lab's most favored domain. Although I have never heard the knowledge engineers themselves articulate this, another consequence of working in scientific domains is that it ensures that they work with experts who are very like themselves.

## The Knowledge Acquisition Problem

From an anthropological standpoint, knowledge acquisition involves a complex sequence of tasks. Not only must the knowledge engineer understand the expert's decision-making process, itself no trivial task, but that information must then be put into machine-usable form. The sequence requires knowledge engineers to undertake two distinct translations. First, they must construct a model of what the expert does, combining understanding of the expert's explicit model with tacit knowledge and contextual information that the expert may not have articulated. Second, the model constructed by the knowledge engineer must then be translated into the language and categories of a particular computer environment in such a way that the information can be used to generate useful statements about the external world.

Not surprisingly (from the standpoint of a social scientist), knowledge acquisition is often problematic. Scientists at the Lab complain that this task is time-consuming, inefficient, and frustrating for expert and knowledge engineer alike. It has become conventional in the field to refer to it as a "bottleneck" in the process of building expert systems (Buchanan, Barstow, Bechtal, Bennett, Clancey, Kulikowski, Mitchell, and Waterman 1983: 129), and a substantial literature has arisen about the so-called "knowledge acquisition problem." The following quotations from that literature illustrate the knowledge engineers' sense of frustration:

> Knowledge acquisition is sometimes considered a necessary burden, carried out under protest so that one can get on with the study of cognitive processes in problem solving (Stefik and Conway 1982: 4).

> Collecting and encoding the knowledge needed to build an ITS [intelligent tutoring system] is still a long and difficult task, and substantial project resources must still be allocated to this stage. Of course, the lack of good high-level tools for knowledge acquisition is a serious problem (Miller 1988: 180).

Most social scientists would probably expect knowledge acquisition to pose a problem. From our perspective, it is a formidable task to gather and order human expertise so completely and so explicitly as to enable a computer to apply it. Those who have written about expert systems have generally been distinctly skeptical about the entire project of automating human intelligence.[13] In one sense, then, social scientists and knowledge engineers can be said to be in agreement that there is a knowledge acquisition problem. However, they often have very different ideas about just what that problem is.[14]

When confronting the idea of expert systems, social scientists tend to focus on the nature of knowledge. Those who have written about such systems would probably agree on the following points. First, knowledge is socially and culturally constituted (Geertz 1973, 1983). Second, knowledge is not self-evident: it must be interpreted. Messages are seen as having meaning because the interlocutors share knowledge about the world (Collins, Green, and Draper 1985; Suchman 1987). Third, people are not completely aware of everything they know: a good deal of knowledge is tacit (Polanyi 1965). Fourth, much knowledge is not in people's heads at all, but is rather "distributed through the division of labor, the procedures for getting things done, etc."[15] Fifth, the relation between what people think they do, what they say they do, and what they can be observed to do is highly complex (Collins 1985; Geertz 1973, 1983). And sixth, because of all these points, complete and unambiguous knowledge about expert procedures is unlikely to be transmitted through experts' verbal or written self-reports (Collins 1985, 1987b; Suchman 1987).

Knowledge engineers see the knowledge acquisition problem quite differently. From their standpoint, the difficulty is not in the nature of knowledge or in the limitations of knowledge elicitation procedures based exclusively on experts' verbal reports.[16] Rather, as one Lab member explained, the difficulty is that "human beings are involved in the loop" and humans are inefficient. The solution, according to the knowledge engineers, will be to automate knowledge acquisition.

> The bottleneck concerns getting the known volume of information into a computer representation, not in getting yet more information out of experts. For example, if we could have textbooks automatically translated into computer representations maybe 80 percent of the perceived bottleneck would be resolved.[17]

This perspective seems to be widely shared at the Lab and is widespread in the AI literature as well.

> This knowledge is currently acquired in a very painstaking way; individual computer scientists work with individual experts to explicate the experts' heuristics—to mine those jewels of knowledge out of their heads one by one. If applied AI is to be important in the decades to come—and we believe it is— we must develop more automatic means for what is currently a very tedious, time-consuming, and expensive procedure (Feigenbaum and McCorduck 1984: 85).

> Automating the knowledge acquisition process can avoid the "Feigenbaum bottleneck" of information between the knowledge engineer and domain expert.[18]

Social scientists tend to see the process of knowledge acquisition as inherently difficult. In contrast, AI people clearly believe that it can be done much more efficiently and look forward to the day when automation will accomplish this goal. This difference in perspective reflects a divergence in what one might call disciplinary worldview: knowledge engineers operate on the basis of some values and assumptions that are quite different from those of social scientists.

## VALUES AND ASSUMPTIONS OF KNOWLEDGE ENGINEERS

In this section I explore some of the values and assumptions that are shared by knowledge engineers at the Lab and that seem to have a bearing on their approach to knowledge acquisition. This material relates to two levels: first, the knowledge engineers' personal and interactional style; and second, their style of thought as scientists. Although for organizational reasons I attempt to separate these categories, in reality they are closely interwoven.

The knowledge engineers at the Lab are not homogeneous. On the contrary, there are some noticeable philosophical and behavioral differences among them. For example, one division in the Lab is that between the so-called "neats" and "scruffies," terms used by my informants to characterize people who engage in different styles of AI research. "Neats" prefer an approach characterized by formal logic, quantitative methods, and the assumption of perfect certainty, whereas "scruffies" prefer to rely on heuristics, qualitative methods, and reasoning with uncertainty. (These categories actually break down further. For example, there are "certain" and "uncertain" neats.) Although Lab members vary in the position they take on the neat/scruffy question, the Lab is generally associated with the scruffy position. Some scruffies express rivalry or antagonism toward neats, criticizing the latter as "not doing AI"; neats in turn criticize scruffies as "inexact" and "unscientific."

Despite such internal diversity, the Lab unquestionably "feels" different from, say, an anthropology department. One reason is that Lab members share some distinctive assumptions and practices. Compared with anthropologists, they have different notions about what a problem is, and of what can be a problem; given a problem, they tend to approach it differently and have different ideas about what counts as evidence. Although neither anthropology nor knowledge engineering constitutes an entire culture, such differences in approach between them can validly be called cultural.

## The "Culture" of Knowledge Engineering: Personal Style

There is an ongoing debate in the field about whether AI is "really" science or engineering (ch. 6; Partridge 1987). Observation suggests that in a sense it is both: my informants tend to define themselves as scientists but often seem to approach things in ways that suggest popular stereotypes of engineers (see below).

### Self-Definition as Scientists

The Lab's researchers are positivists who describe themselves as scientists. They have backgrounds in such fields as engineering, computer science, chemistry, medicine, and cognitive science. One or two are also trained in mathematics, physics, and/or philosophy; none has a background in sociology or cultural anthropology.

Both neats and scruffies at the Lab seem concerned to establish AI as a science, although they have rather different agendas for the development of the discipline. Perhaps because they see themselves as inventing a new field whose identity they feel a need to protect, the Lab's knowledge engineers (especially scruffies) seem reluctant to borrow from other disciplines. Those who do so are liable to criticism for "not doing AI." While this attitude may help to establish the disciplinary boundaries of their new science, it also leads knowledge engineers in some cases to reinvent the wheel (ch. 6). As we shall see, one example of this is knowledge elicitation methodology.

*Engineering Ethos*

In apparent contrast with their self-identification with science, people at the Lab share a style expressive of what I call an "engineering ethos." This has a number of aspects, but perhaps the most salient is the technical orientation of the Lab members. There are two sides to this. On the one hand, they are inclined to think of technical matters as posing interesting problems. In contrast, social matters are not conceived of as problematic in an important way. This is not to suggest that social phenomena may not be *troublesome*—indeed, they often are, as in the case of knowledge elicitation—but they are not thought of as interesting. Categorized as "a matter of common sense," social phenomena fall outside the category of unsolved problems that knowledge engineers like to think about. This view was illustrated by a Lab member who compared detailed discussion of interview methodology with "telling adults how to tie their shoes." The other side of this is that when problems are recognized to occur, they are likely to be assumed to be technical in nature and to require a technical solution.

A second aspect of this "engineering ethos" is a tendency to approach things practically rather than theoretically. Faced with a problem, the Lab's knowledge engineers prefer to try to solve it in a rough and ready way, refining the solution by trial and error. When building an expert system, they say, it is better build a rapid prototype and see how it turns out than to map it out exhaustively beforehand. As one Lab member explained, "If you waited to figure out what you were doing, you'd never get anything done. There just isn't time to do that." He characterized the general approach (ironically) as "Let's not stop to think, let's just do it and we'll find out." Performance is the criterion here. Lab people assume that the first version of a system will have to be thrown away and that the inadequacies of the prototype will be obvious. I have never heard anyone at the Lab address in detail the question of how to evaluate a system built in this way or how to ensure that the second version will be better than the first.

This action-oriented style applies on other levels as well. For example, asked to define "artificial intelligence," some knowledge engineers respond that they do not know what AI is. Rather than debate about the definition of "intelligence," or discuss whether AI is or is not part of computer science, they prefer to get on with their systems.

And finally, some of the knowledge engineers have a rather shy or introverted style of social interaction. While they may be friendly, they do not always seem to find it easy to communicate in a face-to-face setting, especially one that is unfamiliar. They give the impression of preferring computers to people, perhaps because computers are less demanding and more predictable than humans (Edwards 1990: 109–10). Speaking of the knowledge engineer on a joint project, one expert commented: "Engineers by and large have dreadful communication skills. One can succeed in technical fields without these skills."

## The "Culture" of Engineering Knowledge: Intellectual Style

Having attempted to characterize something of the Lab members' personal style, I turn now to the question of their intellectual style. Below I consider two themes, which both relate to the material above and shape my informants' approach to the knowledge acquisition problem. These are the Lab members' tendency to reify knowledge and their view of face-to-face data collection as a commonsense procedure.

### Reification of Knowledge

One of the researchers at the Lab is fond of repeating Feigenbaum's "knowledge principle," which asserts that "In the knowledge is the power" (Feigenbaum and McCorduck 1984). This expresses the heuristic that the size and quality of an expert system's knowledge base are the most important factors in determining the level of its performance (Lenat and Feigenbaum 1987: 1173–74). What do the knowledge engineers mean by "knowledge"?

As we have seen, they divide knowledge into "expertise" and "common sense"; conventionally they have assumed that an expert system should encode the former. Occasional pieces of "commonsense" knowledge have had to be added to knowledge bases, as in the medical diagnosis system that had to be told that men do not get pregnant (see below). However, knowledge engineers do not normally set out to collect commonsense knowledge during knowledge elicitation sessions.

In the past decade, however, some AI researchers have come to the conclusion that commonsense knowledge would enable expert systems to deal with much broader domains (Lenat and Feigenbaum 1987; McCarthy 1984). A research group led by Douglas Lenat is now engaged in a major project designed to collect such knowledge. Rather than investigating what constitutes common sense in particular cases or contexts, however, their approach is to try to produce a generalized commonsense database by essentially automating an encyclopedia. (Hence the project name "CYC.") In addition to entering in that knowledge base the facts cited in the encyclopedia, knowledge engineers on the project are asked to introspect about and enter in the system all the information they believe is needed to understand each encyclopedia entry (Guha and Lenat 1990; Lenat and Guha 1990; Lenat, Prakash, and Shepherd 1986).

This project illustrates two aspects of the way in which AI researchers seem to think about knowledge. First, "knowledge" tends to be understood to mean formal or codified knowledge such as that contained in encyclopedias and textbooks. "What everybody knows" is less likely to be treated as knowledge. This contrasts with the anthropological view of knowledge (including common sense) as cultural (Geertz 1973, 1983). Second, people in AI rely a good deal on introspection as a method of research. Faced with a statement about the nature of human intelligence, my informants evaluate it not by seeking out empirical data (as an anthropologist would) but rather by introspecting. Having found a statement to apply to them, they appear willing to accept that it applies to human beings in general. I have come to think of this style of thought as "I am the world" reasoning.

Knowledge engineers talk about knowledge as though it were something concrete. As the term "knowledge acquisition" implies, they seem to view it as a straightforward, bounded entity that can intentionally be acquired. This is illustrated in the language with which knowledge acquisition is discussed, both at the Lab and in the literature. For example, one Lab member asserted in a lecture that "extracting . . . knowledge from an expert's brain can be slow, cumbersome, and very expensive." A textbook defines knowledge acquisition as "the process of extracting, organizing, and structuring knowledge for use in knowledge-based systems" (Boose 1986: 23). And a journal survey article on the topic is entitled "Extracting Expertise from Experts: Methods for Knowledge Acquisition" (Olson and Rueter 1987). The word common to these quotations is "extraction," a word used frequently in connection with knowledge acquisition. For knowledge engineers, knowledge is apparently a "thing" that can be extracted, like a mineral or a diseased tooth.[19]

When we look further at the language that knowledge engineers use, this impression is reinforced. The survey article mentioned above describes a number of methods for "getting the knowledge out of the expert and into the system" (Olson and Rueter 1987: 152). According to the text, knowledge can be "acquired," "uncovered," "revealed," "cloned," "elicited," and "stored" (Olson and Rueter 1987: 153–67). Knowledge is portrayed here as a structured, stable entity. It is apparently believed to be structured in the expert's brain according to the same principles that structure an expert system: "Experts have stored rich representations of facts, objects and their attributes, as well as a set of inference rules that connect constellations of facts for use in problem-solving situations" (ibid., p. 166). However, getting hold of this knowledge requires effort, since it must be uncovered, revealed, or elicited.

Knowledge engineers, then, seem to think of knowledge elicitation as a sort of surgical or engineering task, in which the substrate to be mined or operated upon is a human brain. They understand this process as a matter of information transfer, not of the construction or translation of knowledge (as a social scientist would tend to think of it).

### Commonsense View of Methodology

Now I turn to the knowledge engineers' attitude toward knowledge elicitation methodology. Informants at the Lab have repeatedly assured me of the unproblematic nature of knowledge elicitation. As one said, "Knowledge elicitation is quite a standard science." Another commented, "We know how to do knowledge acquisition."

People at the Lab do not seem to think of face-to-face knowledge elicitation as calling for any special theory or methodology.[20] On the contrary, they view it as a simple matter of talking to experts and finding out what they know. Asked how he went about this process, for example, one senior Lab member said, "Oh, that's just a matter of common sense." The issues of how to talk with experts, how to get them to articulate the knowledge that constitutes their expertise, how to obtain knowledge that they cannot articulate, and how to understand and record that information do not seem to strike my informants as requiring discussion. Questions on these topics tend to produce blank stares of incomprehension. From their standpoint, it seems that the gathering of human expertise is both conceptually and methodologically straightforward.

However, they do not necessarily enjoy the process; indeed, they appear to do their best to avoid it. Lab members use several tactics to minimize the amount of face-to-face interviewing they have to do for knowledge elicitation. First, it is conventional at the Lab to use only one expert per system. The knowledge engineers explain that it is very difficult to get experts to agree about anything. Since a project with multiple experts is bound to require the knowledge engineer to mediate between them, this is best avoided. The single-expert policy keeps the knowledge engineers from having to make contact with a large number of informants. Second, the more senior Lab members avoid doing knowledge elicitation by assigning the job to junior people. On the projects I have observed, much of the interviewing was carried out by graduate students. Third, knowledge engineers at the Lab prefer if possible to use themselves as experts. Rather than have to interview anyone, they gravitate toward expert systems projects that allow them to construct their own knowledge bases through introspection. And fourth, where systems are built that require the knowledge engineer to carry out knowledge elicitation using experts other than themselves, people at the Lab show a preference for subject areas that are already highly codified, such as medicine. This allows them to obtain a good deal of the knowledge base from written materials and presumably also facilitates the communicative tasks involved in the knowledge elicitation itself.

Why do the Lab members try to avoid face-to-face knowledge elicitation? After all, given their own view of knowledge acquisition as simple information transfer, the process shouldn't be a problem. I suggest that several things account for this. First, as the knowledge engineers point out, knowledge elicitation is time-consuming. A social scientist would expect this to be so because of the nature of the task; defining the task differently, the knowledge engineers perceive knowledge elicitation as extremely inefficient. Second, the knowledge engineers' naive approach to knowledge and its elicitation seem to prevent them from anticipating methodological difficulties that might worry a social scientist. However, knowledge elicitation still requires a great deal of face-to-face interaction with an expert. As we saw earlier, knowledge engineers are computer aficionados whose range of communication skills sometimes seems a bit limited. I suggest that some may be uncomfortable at the prospect of extended interaction with a high-status expert—especially under conditions in which there is an obvious measure of their own performance (the future expert system).

This line of reasoning is supported by my own observations of knowledge elicitation sessions. As I have discussed elsewhere (Forsythe and Buchanan 1989), knowledge engineers quite frequently encounter problems of communication in the course of their interviews. When such problems occur, they are not very well equipped to deal with them. Not only may the interactional situation be difficult for them on a personal level, but they have almost certainly had no training in how to conduct an interview. The extensive literature on the knowledge acquisition problem contains little mention of the fact that interviewing is a challenging task that improves with training and practice (Forsythe and Buchanan 1989). Furthermore, the knowledge engineers seem to have no theoretical apparatus for usefully analyzing the conceptual puzzles that are bound to arise during knowledge elicitation. Given their technical training and orientation and their lack of exposure to the social sciences, they approach the process of knowledge elicitation naively, expecting simply to "acquire" the expert's knowledge. When this turns out to be difficult, novice knowledge engineers at least appear baffled. Ironically, knowledge elicitation is probably made more difficult by their expectation that it will be straightforward. If they defined it as an important problem and devoted substantial effort to theoretical and methodological preparation for it, they might well find the actual process easier because they would probably go about it differently.

If the knowledge engineers find knowledge elicitation difficult, what about the domain experts? The extraction imagery certainly implies that experts may not enjoy the process. Both at the Lab and in reports from the literature (e.g., Hill 1986), this expectation seems to be borne out: knowledge engineers do sometimes encounter trouble persuading their experts to cooperate with the process. Observation suggests several reasons for this. Here I will mention two. First, knowledge engineers—especially men—tend to define the situation in a purely task-oriented way: the expert is there to have his brain mined, not to engage in social niceties. Asked about interactional aspects of his own knowledge elicitation sessions, for example, one knowledge engineer replied that worrying about such things was a luxury for which he was too busy. He characterized as "prima donnas" people who became offended by "rough and ready" individuals like him.

> In the beginning I was paying attention to whether I was offending [my expert], but now I've stopped thinking about it. . . . If I run up against someone who's a prima donna, I figure it's their problem, not mine.

Experts may not enjoy this rather instrumental approach. One said of a young knowledge engineer, "He treated me like a dog!" Second, the knowledge engineers' commonsense approach to interviewing is sometimes rather haphazard. Experts as well as interviewers become frustrated by the sense that they do not know where the process is going. Convinced that the expert's interest will be rekindled when an actual system is produced, knowledge engineers may simply push on rather than taking the time to discuss the situation.

When problems do occur during knowledge elicitation, they are often blamed on the expert. Knowledge engineers attribute these problems to such factors as presumed psychological difficulties on the part of the experts. According to one knowledge engineer, "Experts are a cantankerous lot." Another stated categorically that all members of the public are "computerphobic." And a textbook on knowledge acquisition offers the following warning:

> A more difficult problem arises if the expert develops a subconscious hostility or fear. This will mean that he fails to provide the correct information even when he is seeming to cooperate (Hart 1986: 46).

Like many aspects of the Lab members' approach to knowledge elicitation, these comments recall the engineering ethos described earlier. They reflect the knowledge engineers' emphasis on action rather than reflection, their definition of interesting problems as those involving technical matters, and their discomfort with the uncontrollable nature of social interaction.

DISCUSSION

For purposes of discussion, I turn now to some more general comments about the knowledge engineers' understanding of "knowledge" and its implications for the way they go about building intelligent systems. Star (1989) has pointed out that scientific practice is a form of work. Building upon

Strauss's insight that "work is the link between the visible and the invisible," she describes the work of translating visible, material reality into "clean, docile" abstractions (Star 1991: 265). As we have seen, knowledge acquisition involves representing complex social and material processes as abstract rules for the knowledge base of an expert system. Thus, in one sense, it constitutes straightforward work in the sense described by Star—the translation of action and descriptions of action into abstractions encoded in the knowledge base of an expert system. However, this work is also illuminated by turning Star's conception around: in another sense, knowledge engineers try to make the invisible visible, by turning knowledge into computer code. Knowledge engineering requires that the knowledge engineer not only understand a body of information, but also make it so explicit that it can be translated into machine-executable statements. Thus, knowledge must quite literally be rendered visible.

Star draws our attention to what she terms "deletions" in scientific (and other) practice, that is, instances in which particular pieces or types of work are rendered invisible (1991: 265). Knowledge engineers' conception of their task as knowledge transfer represents a significant case of deletion, since the notion of straightforward transfer completely obscures their own role in the selection and interpretation of what goes into a knowledge base. In my view, knowledge engineering is much better seen as a process of construction or translation, since selection and interpretation are intrinsic to the task. As I try to show in this chapter, this task both reflects and requires a particular view of knowledge. If you hold this view of knowledge, the idea of expert systems seems both possible and desirable; if you do not, it may seem to be neither.

## Meaning of "Knowledge"

Drawing on my ethnographic material, I want to list explicitly some of the assumptions that make up the knowledge engineers' (largely tacit) notion of knowledge. In order to characterize their perspective, I will set up an ideal type called "knowledge engineer" and contrast it with another ideal type called "social scientist." Obviously, these are simplifications: knowledge engineers do not all think identically, nor do social scientists. The views I attribute to the former are a distillation of what I have seen as a participant-observer in the world of AI; the views I attribute to the latter clearly reflect my own perspective as an interpretive anthropologist.

1. For knowledge engineers, the nature of knowledge is apparently not problematic. I have never heard a knowledge engineer puzzle about what "knowledge" means, and they tend to react with impatience when I do so. In contrast, social scientists tend to think of knowledge as highly problematic.

2. To knowledge engineers, knowledge is an either/or proposition: it is either present or absent, right or wrong. Knowledge thus seems to be conceived of as an absolute. If you have it, you're an expert; if you lack it, you're a novice. Novices may encounter trouble because some knowledge that they possess is wrong, but this isn't really knowledge. In contrast, social scientists are more likely to believe that we are all experts in some areas and novices in others; and furthermore, that what counts as knowledge is not only highly situational but is also a matter of perspective and cultural background (Geertz 1973: ch. 1; 1983: ch. 4). From this standpoint, knowledge is more usefully thought of in terms of potential and negotiated relevance, rather than as present or absent in any straightforward way.

3. Knowledge engineers seem to conceive of reasoning as a matter of following formal rules. In contrast, social scientists—especially anthropologists—tend to think of it in terms of meaning and to note that the logic by which people reason may differ according to social and cultural context.

4. Knowledge engineers treat knowledge as a purely cognitive phenomenon. Knowledge, to them, is located solely in the individual mind; expertise, then, is a way of thinking. This contrasts with the social scientific view of knowledge as also being encoded in the cultural, social, and organizational order. Given the latter view, contextual factors are seen to play a role in expertise, and knowledge appears to be a social and cultural phenomenon as well as a cognitive one.

5. Knowledge engineers tend to assume that knowledge is conscious, that is, that experts can tell you what they know if only they will. They do not have systematic procedures for exploring tacit knowledge, nor do they seem aware of the inevitably partial nature of the retrospective reporting conventionally used for knowledge elicitation. Textbooks warn knowledge engineers that experts may not tell them everything they need to know, but tend to explain this as lack of cooperation or even as dishonesty on the part of the expert. In contrast, social scientists expect some knowledge to be partially accessible, and some to be inaccessible to the conscious mind. It is for this reason that anthropologists and qualitative sociologists make

extensive use of participant observation for data-gathering purposes, rather than relying upon interview data alone.

6. Knowledge engineers assume that thought and action are isomorphic. Hearing experts' conscious models of their own behavior, they assume that their practice will always or at least usually correspond to them. This is surely one reason that they tend to talk to experts but rarely watch them at work. To social scientists, on the other hand, the relation between belief and action is highly problematic. If anything, anthropologists at least tend to assume that thought and practice are not related in a simple way (Geertz 1973: ch. 1; 1983: ch. 4).

7. And finally, the knowledge engineers seem to think of knowledge as universal. That is, they see it as consisting of "rules" that will apply across contexts. For example, Lenat and colleagues assert that "to build CYC, we must encode all the world's knowledge down to some level of detail; there is no way to finesse this" (Lenat, Prakash, and Shepherd 1986: 75). Given this assumption about the universal nature of knowledge, information that is clearly situational in nature or is only locally applicable may not strike them as knowledge at all. Social scientists, in contrast, place much more emphasis on the significance of local and situational knowledge and on the importance of combining local and global knowledge.[21] (For example, consider the amount of knowledge one needs to possess beforehand in order to do anything with an expert system.)

In short, to knowledge engineers, "knowledge" means explicit, globally applicable rules whose relation to each other and to implied action is straightforward. Knowledge in this sense is a stable entity that can be acquired and transferred. It can be rendered machine-readable and manipulated by a computer program. I believe that in effect "knowledge" has been operationally redefined in AI to mean "what can be programmed into the knowledge base of an expert system."

Star has commented that computer scientists "delete the social."[22] I would add that they delete the cultural as well. These twin deletions characterize every level of knowledge engineering. Of particular relevance to the concerns of this paper, the social and the cultural are deleted from these scientists' concept of knowledge. The AI community has succeeded in automating the AI conception of knowledge. In contrast, it is difficult to imagine how one could automate the alternative that I have called the social science conception of knowledge. In this view, knowledge does not remain stable over time, but is both culturally contingent and reconstructed with changes of time, person, and context. If knowledge is not a constant entity, but rather the outcome of ongoing processes of construction and interpretation, then what should go into a knowledge base of an expert system?

## How This View of Knowledge Affects Expert Systems

Traweek (1988a) has shown that the values of high-energy physicists are embedded in the machines they construct. In the same way, I suggest, the view of knowledge shared by knowledge engineers is encoded in their own expert systems. I will consider four aspects of this.

First, the knowledge in such systems is static. In everyday life, the beliefs held by individuals are modified through negotiation with other individuals; as ideas and expectations are expressed in action, they are also modified in relation to contextual factors. But the information encoded in a knowledge, base is not modified in this way. Knowledge engineers do not normally seek to encode negotiated, situational, or organizational aspects of knowledge, or to set up mechanisms within systems which could themselves negotiate. Just how possible it would be to do such things I do not know; as far as I know, few people have tried. My point is that whereas an anthropologist would regard these points as significant drawbacks in the "knowledge" encoded in an expert system, knowledge engineers generally do not see an omission here at all. When they do take my point that information is being left out, they respond that such information isn't "relevant."

Second, the knowledge in expert systems is brittle. One cause of this is that knowledge engineers generally do not undertake the systematic comparisons between belief and action, or between the views of different experts that would aid them in uncovering tacit knowledge. A famous example of such an omission was provided by MYCIN, one of the first medical diagnostic systems. Given a male patient with a bacterial infection, MYCIN suggested that one likely source of infection might be a prior amniocentesis (Buchanan and Shortliffe 1984: 692). While this is absurd, no one had thought to build into the system's knowledge base the information that men do not get pregnant. Therefore, it did not prune "amniocentesis" from the menu of possible sources of infection in men. Information about where babies come from is representative of a large class of knowledge that experts might not think to explain to knowledge engineers, but which is clearly essential for correct inference in certain areas of human activity. Without such taken-for-granted background knowledge about the world, expert systems tend to "fall off the knowledge cliff" (Davis 1989).

Third, the knowledge in expert systems is narrow, again in part because of the practice of interviewing only one expert. This is illustrated by the history of a well-known system for geological exploration. Initially, the system was built using one expert whose experience was limited to one geographical area of the world. When applied outside this area, the system foundered: since the expert's knowledge was to some extent local, the system could not be applied globally. Apparently this limitation had not occurred to the system developers, who seem to have expected "knowledge" to apply in every context. When the system was later rebuilt using multiple experts with experience in different areas, it was more successful.[23]

I have tried to show how the knowledge engineers' view of knowledge affects the way they define their work, the way in which they go about that work, and the products of that work. Finally, I want to point out that this view of knowledge also shapes their plans for future research. The Lab members look forward to the day when automated knowledge acquisition will eliminate the need for them to interview experts in order to build knowledge-based systems. They believe that automation will get around the knowledge acquisition problem. From the perspective of knowledge engineers, "getting the humans out of the loop" will increase the efficiency and precision of knowledge elicitation by eliminating the ambiguities of face-to-face communication. From a social scientific standpoint, however, this is highly questionable. To rely on automation to solve the knowledge acquisition problem is to propose a technical solution for problems that in my view are largely non-technical. These problems derive in large part from the nature of knowledge. They also stem from the complexities of communication in general and of communication about knowledge in particular, and from certain attributes of the knowledge engineers themselves, including the approach they take to knowledge elicitation and the values and assumptions that underlie that approach.

CONCLUSION

In conclusion, I will relate this ethnographic material to some broader issues. As we have seen, building a knowledge-based system necessarily involves selection and interpretation: Lenat's view notwithstanding (see above), one cannot encode all the world's knowledge. A given knowledge base can contain only some of the available material and encode only a small number of perspectives out of many possible ways of viewing a particular domain. Thus, selectivity is an inevitable aspect of knowledge engineering.

I suggested above that some of the problematic characteristics of current expert systems can be related to the specific notion of knowledge held by the knowledge engineers. This implies that the narrowness and brittleness of expert systems might be ameliorated to some extent if knowledge engineers held a different definition of knowledge, which might in turn lead them to change the methods by which they design and build such systems. Given the overlap between the work of knowledge elicitation and the data-gathering goals of cultural anthropology and qualitative sociology, I believe that it would be helpful to knowledge engineers if their education routinely included some training in the theory and methodology of qualitative social science. By providing them with additional ways of thinking about and carrying out knowledge elicitation, this might assist knowledge engineers to meet their own goal of system-building.

However, teaching social science to knowledge engineers would not eliminate the problem of the selectivity of the knowledge in expert systems. No matter how many experts are used, no matter how expertly they are interviewed and their work practice analyzed, building an expert system still requires human beings to look at a piece of the world, interpret it, and represent their interpretation in the system. I offer three concluding points about this state of affairs.

First, as Bourdieu (1977: 165) has pointed out, the ability to decide what will count as knowledge in a particular case is a form of power. In undertaking the selection and interpretation involved in designing and constructing expert systems, knowledge engineers exercise this type of power. Some decisions concerning knowledge base construction take place quite explicitly: knowledge engineers are aware that they have to make choices about what to include in their systems. However, I argue that decisions about what goes into a knowledge base also occur implicitly, through the application of the knowledge engineers' own tacit values and assumptions. The factor I have focused upon here is their concept of knowledge. The knowledge engineers' particular understanding of knowledge contributes to the selectivity of their knowledge bases in a variety of ways, through such conventions as the practice of interviewing only one expert per system or that of structuring knowledge elicitation around the search for formal rules. Such implicit consequences of taken-for-granted meanings illustrate the cultural nature of scientific practice.

Second, the exercise of this power is to some extent invisible. To begin with, it is clearly invisible to many users of such systems. Design decisions taken by individual knowledge engineers are encoded in computer languages that most people cannot read and embedded in tools that function as (and in some cases quite literally are) black boxes (Latour and Woolgar 1986: 242, 259–60). Once an expert system is built, it is all too easy for the user to take it at face value, assuming that what the system says must be correct. Since most people who use such systems in business, medicine, or the military know little about how they are produced, they may not question the nature of the knowledge they contain. In addition, the power they exercise is at least to some extent invisible to knowledge engineers themselves. Because knowledge-based systems in a sense replicate their makers' perspective, system-builders may not themselves recognize everything that has been tacitly built into a system or what has been excluded from it. This is a small version of the problem of "seeing" one's own culture. Furthermore, while system-builders know that every knowledge base has its limitations, they do not appear to be aware that members of the public may not know this. Possible misunderstandings on the part of future users are not viewed as their problem.

And third, although the knowledge engineers do not think of it this way, the power they exercise has a political aspect (Bourdieu 1977). The design process raises numerous questions about the relationship between technology and society that are routinely deleted from discussion. While the knowledge engineers would probably label such questions philosophical, they have important cultural and political dimensions. For example, when an expert system is built, whose interpretation of reality should it encode? Whose "knowledge" should constitute the "knowledge base"; whose practice should be enshrined as "expertise"? Only a small number of training cases and/or a finite amount of knowledge can be accommodated by an individual system. So who should select the cases or the "knowledge" that will stand for "reality"? How representative are these selections, and what do they represent? Whose interests are embedded in that "knowledge"? And what will be done with the "knowledge" in the system? The development of very large knowledge bases designed to be accessed by large numbers of systems makes such questions even more pertinent from a political standpoint, but I have never heard knowledge engineers raise them. Perhaps because they view knowledge as absolute rather than as representing particular interests and perspectives, such questions tend to be swept under the rug in AI.

These deleted questions relate to major political issues concerning differences in culture, race, class, and gender. Many knowledge engineers are white, middle class, Western men; most designated "experts" come from the same background.[24] The knowledge in expert systems inevitably reflects the interests and perspectives of these individuals. It is much less likely to represent the interests and perspectives of individuals from other backgrounds in our increasingly diverse society. Those whose ways of knowing and doing are classified as "knowledge" and "expertise" by the builders of expert systems will find their view of the world reinforced and empowered by this powerful emerging technology. Those whose perspectives and practice are not so classified are likely to find their voices muted still further as the world increasingly relies upon intelligent machines.[25] Thus, Feigenbaum's assertion that "in the knowledge is the power" may apply most strongly in a sense in which he did not intend it—with reference to the power to "engineer" the knowledge that confers the power of expert systems.

# CHAPTER FOUR

# Knowing Engineers? A Response to Forsythe

*James Fleck*


Diana Forsythe's paper "Engineering Knowledge" contains much interesting material and many thought-provoking observations about a particular community of practitioners—"knowledge engineers," members of the expert systems community within AI [artificial intelligence]. In particular, it provides a telling critique in terms of social science interview methodology of the procedures used by those practitioners, especially as regards the process of "knowledge acquisition" (and more specifically the process of "knowledge elicitation")—the attempt to "capture" from experts the basis for their skills and expertise in a form suitable for encoding into so-called "expert systems." In providing this critique, Forsythe offers a promising line of attack which I believe would signally improve the efforts of the expert system practitioners: namely, to consider seriously the interview process as a social transaction in which the two parties negotiate to construct a model of the knowledge at issue. Indeed, such an approach is beginning to emerge—as evidenced by the explicit employment of social scientists, especially anthropologists, for carrying out the knowledge elicitation process, and by the development of more sophisticated understandings of the whole knowledge engineering process pioneered primarily by psychologists (e.g., Hoffman 1992).

Forsythe herself, however, doubts whether the adoption of a social science appreciation would in fact produce any final solution to the "problem of knowledge acquisition," arguing that there is a fundamental flaw in the practitioners' basic approach and goals. This flaw arises from their technically circumscribed way of defining the situation in the first place. They see knowledge purely in terms of logical rules and do not recognize the importance of social transactions or context. In other words, she is arguing that there is a fundamental epistemological disjunction between the expert systems practitioners' frame of understanding and the nature of the situation as

it would be construed by social scientists. More strongly, she is unequivocally saying that the social scientists' view is *right*; it is how the underlying
reality of the situation *should* be understood.

I do not want to get into the debate about the *ultimate* correctness of the
expert systems approach. It is an argument that in different guises is probably as old as human thought, and it has been particularly heated with respect to the field of AI (including recently in *Social Studies of Science*); and
it will undoubtedly run and run.[1]

I am more immediately concerned with some issues arising from the *stance*
adopted in the paper, which I think has compromised Forsythe's analysis.
This stance is implicitly *epistemologically asymmetric*. By assuming the superiority of a particular framework—that of social science—she missed the
opportunity for a more comprehensive, perhaps less comfortable analysis,
which would also reflexively question whether the expert systems area has
anything to teach social scientists.[2] Forsythe's paper provides a trigger for the
discussion of certain points (sharply stated and no doubt exaggerated), which
I think have wider implications for the social analysis of scientific activity
more generally.

EPISTEMOLOGICAL ASYMMETRY

What I am referring to here as an "epistemological asymmetry" consists of
a somewhat complacent certainty about the social science way of thinking
contrasted with a rather belittling view of the capacity and interests of technical people. This underpins a pervasive "us" (social scientists—that is, "civilized human beings") versus "them" ("naive" knowledge engineers and self-
professed positivists—that is, the "primitive savages") view. This partiality
belies the serious anthropological stance, which claims to "attempt to understand what events mean to the people involved" (ch. 3). The explicit use
of phrases such as "from our perspective" (which includes the readers in the
privileged view and excludes those under study) is a questionable means of
soliciting approval, and again reflects partiality. Consider for contrast the
rather different impact of the following putative but possible formulation:

> As knowledge engineers, we are well-equipped with appropriate formal
> calculi for adequately explaining many of the subtleties of problem-solving
> cognition. But unfortunately, social scientists seem to be blind to the expres-
> sive power of our technical apparatus and are prejudiced to see everything in

terms of politics, which in fact only obscures the essential substantive content of the reasoning taking place.[3]

The pervasive "us"/"them" partiality is reinforced by the stereotypical claim that "engineers are more interested in things rather than people"; specifically, in Forsythe's paper: "They give the impression of preferring computers to people, perhaps because computers are less demanding and more predictable than humans" (ch. 3). Behind this patronizing view is the barely stated implication that consequently they, the engineers, are somehow lacking in humanity, as is often expressed by the devastating and dismissive stereotypical "engineers treat people like things." The specific quote selected in Forsythe's paper to illustrate this lack of human sensibility was, in fact: "He treated me like a dog" (ch. 3).

Of course, this is not to say that such stereotypes do not contain any elements of truth. But they certainly selectively over-simplify, and probably say more about the stance of those holding the view than they do about those to whom the views are imputed. In extreme cases such stereotypes can become a form of "racism"—as with the dismissive and pejorative use of the term "techies," which is common today among some social scientists (though not, it should be emphasized, used by Forsythe). I do not think that "us and them" stances help to further analysis of scientific activity, nor do I think that they are a proper part of the anthropological approach. There is also a danger that the invocation of stereotypes can obscure the issues under analysis.

For example, consider the quote cited by Forsythe from a prominent AI text:

> The knowledge is currently acquired in a very painstaking way: individual computer scientists work with individual experts to explicate the experts' heuristics—to mine those jewels of knowledge out of their heads one by one. If applied AI is to be important in the decades to come—and we believe it is— we must develop more automatic means for what is currently a very tedious, time-consuming, and expensive procedure [ch. 3, quoting Fiegenbaum and McCorduck 1984].

This can readily be interpreted as indicating a sophisticated and sensitive awareness of the nature of knowledge, and even of certain tacit aspects, rather than the naive appreciation attributed by Forsythe to expert system practitioners. So too can the quoted terms: "uncovered," "revealed," and "elicited"; the last, in particular—meaning "to draw forth (what is latent or potential); to educe (principles, etc.) from a person" (Murray 1972)—appears to be an admirable term to cover the difficult task of articulating the subtleties of knowledge.

It is one thing to highlight the mentalism espoused by knowledge engineers, but quite another to evaluate such a mentalism as *implicitly* naive, even though it may so seem from a social science viewpoint. Nevertheless, Forsythe is certainly right, I think, in pointing out that expert systems practitioners' lack of appreciation for the social embeddedness of knowledge. This is, indeed, another valuable insight that social scientists have to give to AI people. It is, however, an issue that is probably best directly addressed with respect to detailed empirical examples, rather than asserted in terms of the simple superiority of one disciplinary framework over another. Furthermore, consideration of what social embeddedness might mean for expert systems raises the notion of a "society" of interacting machines, with interesting implications back again to social science, as already explored by Woolgar's query: Why not a sociology of machines (Woolgar 1985)? And are not machines already minimal social actors (or actants) in their own right?[4]

KNOWLEDGE ENGINEERS AND SOCIAL SCIENTISTS

But with respect to other aspects of knowledge, I doubt whether the appreciation developed by AI practitioners is really so irreconcilably different (or incommensurable) from that developed by social scientists. As well as the already-mentioned suggestions for AI from social science, in some respects AI-related work has useful ideas to offer social scientists. The idea of the "procedural embedding of knowledge," popularized by Winograd (1972) in connection with natural language understanding, for instance, is surely one useful mechanism for certain forms of tacit knowledge.

This is not to say that the goals of social scientists and AI practitioners do not differ. In particular, Forsythe's comment that knowledge engineers *reify* knowledge is literally correct—and, again, is a particularly telling empirical and theoretical insight about the development of technology that could be made much more of, rather than cited almost dismissively. For what is technology in general if not a set of specific forms of reification?

With respect to the discussion about the engineering ethos, AI practitioners are surely as entitled to their view that technical matters are interesting, and social phenomena merely a matter of common sense and less interesting, just as much as Forsythe is entitled to an obvious preference (clear prejudice?) for the contrary view. The appropriate anthropological task is to explicate the coherence in and reasons for these contrasting views, not to pass judgment on which is "right" or "better."[5] But again there is a sense that somehow the social scientists' view is preferable and less naive: "the knowledge engineers' naive approach to knowledge and its elicitation seems to prevent them from anticipating methodological problems that might worry a social scientist" (ch. 3).

The interesting point is that knowledge engineers do construe problems differently than social scientists, and they do have their own distinctive methodological concerns, which are related to the instruments employed and their own criteria of procedural efficacy—namely, whether the system does in fact work or not. Such criteria clearly go a long way to explaining the pragmatic approach of "getting on with it" adopted by the knowledge engineers. To explore these questions it would be worthwhile looking at how success and failure are constructed by the practitioners, rather than overplaying the implicit judgments between naive engineers and sophisticated social scientists.

In this connection, Star's notion of "deletion of the social" is a powerful one. However, its expression in Forsythe's paper is another instance where the epistemological asymmetry is evident. I think the metaphor of "deletion," with its negative overtones, is perhaps misplaced. It is not so much a matter of anything being deleted, but rather that certain aspects are focused on and developed (or even constructed), while others are simply not perceived in the first place. Practicing engineers do not so much wantonly destroy the social,[6] as *inflate* the technical; they construe the world in terms of their own cognitive resources and constructs. As Kuhn pointed out, technical paradigms or frameworks of understanding have a powerful focusing aspect which directs attention to a hitherto small and overlooked part of the world, and thereby drives progressive development (Kuhn 1970).

Certainly, "the social" is not the central concern in the creative interests and discourse of knowledge engineers that it is with social scientists. Knowledge engineers see the world in terms of factual knowledge bases, procedural rules ("production systems") and software mechanisms (including "inference engines"), which meet particular technical criteria of adequacy and efficacy, associated with the computational instruments used. These terms differ from those used by social scientists, as does the focus of interest. By focusing on the procedurally explicable in such terms, knowledge engineers thereby "inflate the technical."

However, by following a reductionist (to social scientists) heuristic in pursuit of what is computationally expressible, they are in any case going to throw more light on the nature of knowledge than if they adopted an attitude which essentially accepts the phenomena as inexplicable. And I am confident that by pursuing such a research program they will eventually discover for themselves the necessity for, and the limits of, the socially embedded and tacit (that is, non-articulable) aspects of knowledge. I am confident because I am convinced, as a social scientist, about the reality of such aspects. To put it another way, expert systems work provides us with a ready-made laboratory in which the essential requirements for tacit knowledge and the like are made apparent by exhausting what can be done with the explicable.[7]

## A BROADER PERSPECTIVE

Standing back, therefore, we can see that what we have here are two broad approaches to the nature of knowledge. *Both* areas of expertise—social science and expert systems—have their own frames of conception and interpretation which selectively expand and create certain aspects of the worlds they respectively inhabit, and simply do not perceive others—that is, they "delete" them. It is peculiarly incumbent upon us, as social analysts of scientific knowledge, to be sensitive to our own lacunae of perception. The "deletion of the social" among engineers and scientists can arguably be balanced against an equivalent "deletion of the technical," prevalent among many social scientists. And a particular danger for social studies of science analysts is that, if taken too far, the "deletion of the technical" may represent an all-too-attractive retreat into the shelter of disciplinary purity, and away from an early commitment in the field to explore precisely how the social and technical are related (as discussed by many, including Whitley 1972).

Meta-epistemological guidelines may help for understanding how very different disciplinary frameworks can clash or merge. This is particularly important for social studies of science, which have a direct interest in examining the development of other bodies of practice. The comprehensive elaboration of such guidelines is obviously a large and continuing challenge, but I would suggest some essential minimal elements may be readily identified. Those pursuing social studies of science should avoid the *unquestioning* imposition of their own values, epistemology, methods, or techniques on the areas they seek to analyze. Anthropological impartiality and epistemological symmetry (especially evaluative neutrality), along with other symmetries advocated in social studies of science and technology,[8] would appear to be suitable starting elements. The opening up of broader channels of communication through the institution of collaborative research (as suggested by several participants in the *Social Studies of Science* Symposium on AI),[9] is another programmatic suggestion. However, precisely because of the enculturational learning processes inevitably involved in such endeavors, this is generally a much longer term proposition.

There has always been a substantial degree of incommensurability and even antipathy between social science and science and engineering, with no prospect for a neat and tidy consensual synthesis. But there certainly *can* be two-way communication (we[10] are all human beings!), and if strenuous attempts are made to be impartial, this may occasionally lead to creative developments in both frames of analysis.

# CHAPTER FIVE

# STS (Re)constructs Anthropology: Reply to Fleck

Fleck's comments on "Engineering Knowledge" (ch. 3) present me with a challenge that is familiar and often frustrating to cultural anthropologists: trying to discuss meanings constructed within a relativist framework with someone who talks like a positivist.[1] The central problem is that statements framed within one perspective are understood and interpreted quite differently from within the other, leading to communicative difficulties that are in a small sense cultural. Relativists talk comfortably on the paradigmatic level; positivists may not. Statements about paradigmatic differences may strike the latter as a put-down, whereas to the relativist they constitute simple description. Although Fleck is not (I take it) a knowledge engineer, he appears to identify with them and to share at least some elements of my informants' worldview. This produces the nicely reflexive consequence that the Fleck-Forsythe exchange replicates the epistemological disjunction that is the subject of my paper.

However, my pleasure at this turn of events is diminished considerably by Fleck's hostile tone. He is extremely reactive to anything that (to him) smacks of "devastating and dismissive stereotyp[es]" of technical people, which he describes as "a form of 'racism.'" This leads him to interpret my description of the differing perspectives of anthropologists and knowledge engineers as an attack on the latter—and also (apparently) as a personal attack on him. In attempting to "defend" my informants and himself against what was of course never intended as an attack on anyone, he misreads my text as well as my motivation in writing it. However, the tone of Fleck's response seems unreasonable, since I am perfectly up front in the paper that I am not a knowledge engineer, that I see the latter from an anthropological standpoint, and that my intent is to describe and characterize their practice in terms of my own perspective.

Fleck frames as matters of fact things that I view as interpretations reflecting our divergent perspectives. For example, what he interprets as "belittling . . . technical people" and showing "a fundamental lack of insight into technical practice" are from my standpoint simply descriptions of things from a different perspective from his.[2] Although Fleck does not address matters on this level, I suggest that most of his substantive criticisms arise from a paradigm clash: we take very different things for granted about social science, about anthropology, and about the nature of knowledge. Thus, Fleck's critique provides a beautiful demonstration of exactly what I was talking about in the paper: the tacit assumptions characteristic of different scientific disciplines affect the attribution of meaning in a way that can validly be called "cultural."

Fleck criticizes me for not doing things that I did not set out to do (see below) and takes me to task for "unequivocally saying" things that I did not say. To illustrate the latter, he correctly summarizes my paper as "arguing that there is a fundamental epistemological disjunction between the expert systems practitioners' frame of understanding and the nature of the situation as it would be construed by social scientists." However, he then goes on to assert, "More strongly, she is unequivocally saying that the social scientists' view is *right*; it is how the underlying reality of the situation *should* be understood." Here Fleck has misunderstood, interpreting my message on the basis of assumptions quite different from those in terms of which it was framed. I do not assert or believe that what I called the social scientists' view is more "right" than that of the knowledge engineers, nor do I believe that there is any single "underlying reality" to the situation. Rather, my point is that the epistemological stance taken by members of two particular disciplinary communities is not the same, and that such epistemological commitments have consequences for the way the members of these communities go about their work. Attempting to understand and describe different collective ways of viewing the world is the fundamental project of cultural anthropology. To notice that truth is constructed quite differently in different human communities is not to denigrate those whose perspective differs from that of the anthropologist. On the contrary, surely respect for other human beings requires that one *not* assume that everyone holds one's own assumptions. My characterization of the disparity between what knowledge engineers and anthropologists take for granted is in no way intended to "belittl[e] . . . the capacity and interests of technical people."

Fleck's reaction to my work is an expression of his own worldview, to which on the whole he is welcome. However, there are two matters on which I wish to take issue with him. First, his perspective on my material seems to lead him to misread the paper in very basic ways. Second, some of his assumptions about anthropology are simply inaccurate. I take up each of these themes below.

## MISREADING THE PAPER

In his written review of my paper for this journal (but a comment not included in his published response), Fleck criticized my "tendency to overgeneralize the empirical material which is based on a restricted study of knowledge engineers in one laboratory." However, the text of the paper states quite clearly that it is based upon field research in five different expert systems laboratories plus considerable professional activity in the wider AI community. It also states that I have been carrying out this field research since 1986. This adds up to a great deal of fieldwork and the accumulation of an enormous amount of data about the practice and the results of knowledge engineering. If at this point I do not have grounds for a certain amount of generalization, I wonder who does. Fleck himself certainly doesn't hold back on this score. Although offering no alternative empirical evidence, his reply generalizes broadly about both knowledge engineers and social scientists.

In a less blatant instance of misreading, Fleck objects repeatedly to what he calls the paper's "pervasive 'us'/'them' partiality." He comments: "The explicit use of phrases such as 'from our perspective' (which includes the readers in the privileged view and excludes those under study) is a questionable means of soliciting approval, and again reflects partiality." Actually, my intent was neither to solicit approval (whose?) nor to include the reader in my view, privileged or not. The phrase "from our perspective" occurs in the context of an explicit comparison between what is taken for granted by knowledge engineers and what is taken for granted by interpretive cultural anthropologists. The "we" intended here is anthropologists, a category to which I belong. Since the paper was written for an STS audience consisting largely of non-anthropologists, the intent of this and similar passages is to present some information about an anthropological perspective to readers from other disciplines. Where Fleck darkly suspects an attempt to enlist the reader in an epistemological conspiracy against knowledge engineers, what

I intended was simply to highlight some different assumptions held by anthropologists and knowledge engineers for the benefit of readers who might not be familiar with either perspective.

## FLECK'S VIEW OF ANTHROPOLOGY

Fleck seems unfamiliar with practices quite standard in anthropology. For example, he does not understand why I do not take my informants' views at face value, as he appears to do. Nor does he distinguish between offering an explicit critique of their practice (which I intend and which is a legitimate anthropological task; see Marcus and Fischer 1986) and patronizing them as people (which I do not intend and would—with Fleck—deplore). Surprisingly, in view of this unfamiliarity, many of his criticisms of "Engineering Knowledge" involve the claim that my work is bad anthropology. Underlying his comments on this theme is a set of tacit assumptions about what he sees as "[t]he appropriate anthropological task." Fleck's willingness to instruct me in my own discipline seems remarkable, although it reflects a certain tendency within STS to appropriate anthropology.[3] Fleck's (unacknowledged) normative beliefs about how anthropology ought to be done define a distinctive perspective from which he examines my performance as fieldworker and writer of anthropological text, and finds it wanting. However, his assumptions correspond to an outdated and discredited notion of anthropology that I do not share. To clarify the difference in our understanding of "the appropriate anthropological task," I offer some background information on my discipline.

### *"Neutrality" and the Problem of Perspective*

Fleck chides me for my lack of "[a]nthropological impartiality," "epistemological symmetry," and "evaluative neutrality." This implies that objectivity is possible for a human observer. If by "evaluative neutrality" Fleck means to suggest freedom from any beliefs and assumptions about the world, then surely this is impossible. All healthy human beings past early childhood have been socialized into a cultural tradition; such traditions encode beliefs and assumptions about the world. Formal education involves further socialization into points of view which differ to some extent by discipline. Humans do not easily set aside an epistemological stance, in part because they tend to be unaware that they hold one. This is the problem of seeing one's own culture to which I refer in my paper. However, one way to become more aware of at least some of what one takes for granted is systematically to investigate the perspective of people who see the world differently. This of course is the task of the field anthropologist; immersed in another cultural setting, fieldwork entails an ongoing attempt to disentangle one's own perspective from that of one's informants.

Anthropologists have long been concerned with the issue of perspective, and with the related problems of relativism and reflexivity. Cultural relativism has been under discussion since the days of Boas and Malinowski, early in this century. Although he did not use this term, Bateson's 1936 experiment (1958) in analytical perspectives addresses some aspects of the issue of reflexivity. Later, the question of voice formed the basis of a disciplinary critique by feminist anthropologists in the 1970s (Morgen 1989), and was widely discussed within the discipline in the 1980s (Geertz 1988; Marcus and Fischer 1986; Rosaldo 1993). By now, the cultural nature of truth and the problematic relationship between observer, observed, and text have received a great deal of attention within anthropology. The positivism of nineteenth- and early twentieth-century anthropologists has long since given way to an acknowledgment that what humans (including social scientists) see in the world has a great deal to do with the assumptions and the conceptual system that they bring to the seeing. These ideas have been much discussed in the recent STS literature as well (Traweek 1988a; Woolgar 1988; Gusterson 1992). Thus, there can be few qualitative social scientists around today who do not find the words "impartiality" and "neutrality" problematic. Seemingly unaffected by all this, Fleck's notion of anthropological objectivity sounds outdated.

What anthropologists aspire to is not "neutrality" but rather *awareness*. Fieldworkers attempt to be conscious not only of the perspectives of their informants, but also of their own point of view. This is why the paper describes my epistemological commitments as well as those of the knowledge engineers. I do this not because I believe that "the social scientists' view is *right*," as Fleck contends, but rather because what I take for granted inevitably influences the way in which I perceive and describe the viewpoint of my informants. I understand my task not as speaking for my informants, as Fleck seems to believe (and which would hardly constitute "impartiality" either), but rather as characterizing for the reader two different perspectives on the problem of knowledge. This approach is by no means restricted to anthropologists of science and technology. Star takes much the same position in her 1989 book. Describing this stance as "the hallmark of sociological analysis" (1989: 19), she writes:

[E]ach way of knowing is accorded a certain integrity based on the recognition that different situations create different perspectives. . . . This is *not* value-neutrality but rather the opposite. As a scientist, I can never be exempt from having a perspective; the sociology is in understanding that everyone else does, too. (Whether I agree or disagree with them is a different question.) (1989: 19).

In sum, the goal of neutrality is Fleck's idea, not mine. In any case, since his generalizations and his perspective on *my* work would be hard to call neutral, he does not seem to adhere to his own standard.

## Does Understanding Require "Going Native"?

Fleck seems disturbed that I do not share the knowledge engineers' epistemological stance, and equates this with bias on my part and a patronizing attitude toward my informants. I suggest that this view implies confusion on *his* part about what anthropologists seek to accomplish by undertaking extended participant observation. The fieldworker's goal is not to adopt the worldview of her informants. To do so is known as "going native" (a term that recalls anthropology's colonial past). Since doing this changes an ethnographer's relationship to her own world as well as that of her informants, it implies a decision to stop field research. On occasion, anthropologists do set aside their research, consciously taking up their informants' point of view in order to engage in political or other action. However, this does not reflect "neutrality," as Fleck suggests, but rather conscious adoption of a *different* perspective.

Viewing the world through the eyes of one's informants is a methodological strategy, not the end of anthropological research. Undertaking participant observation means engaging in a systematic process that Powdermaker calls "stepping in and stepping out" of the field situation (Powdermaker 1966). Moving in both a physical and a cognitive sense back and forth between two sociocultural systems, the fieldworker uses her own experience to become aware of the ways in which these systems are constituted. The first stage of this process ("stepping in") is immersion in the informants' community in order to understand how they view the world and the nature of their practice in it. In my own case, I "stepped in" when in late 1986 I began to spend my working days in an artificial intelligence laboratory, becoming over time an accepted (if somewhat anomalous) member of the Lab. As Fleck implies, a central goal of this stage is indeed to understand how and why one's informants view the world as they do—as I believe I do understand the intellectual perspective of the knowledge engineers with whom I work.

However, if personal immersion is to result in research (as opposed to going native), this first stage must be followed by the second stage of "stepping out" again, back to one's own context. This is necessary in order to acquire enough distance from the field situation to *analyze* it as opposed to simply reporting the views of one's informants. When fieldwork takes place in a distant location, "stepping out" is a physical as well as a cognitive process. When the field site is closer to home, as in a nearby scientific laboratory, the physical stepping out may be largely metaphorical (as it is in my case). Nevertheless, it remains necessary to leave the field site in a cognitive sense: critical analysis depends upon stepping out of the informants' worldview back into one's own intellectual frame of reference.

Far from implying disrespect to the knowledge engineers, my analysis of their practice from a conceptual framework outside their own is part of what constitutes my work as anthropology. I might point out that I have discussed this theme exhaustively with my own informants and have shown them Fleck's comments on my paper as well as the paper itself. In response to Fleck's suggestion that my critical stance toward knowledge engineering practice implies a patronizing attitude, the head of the lab pointed out that it is precisely this critical stance that makes my presence in his work group useful to him.

### Pith Helmets in the Laboratory? Fleck's Colonial View of Anthropology

Fleck describes my paper as portraying social scientists as "civilized human beings" and "naive knowledge engineers and self-professed positivists" as "primitive savages." Depicting my informants as powerless, voiceless victims of a powerful observer, he apparently believes that he is speaking on their behalf. This is absurd. It is Fleck's notion of anthropological fieldwork that contains these colonial images, not mine. His identification with what he takes to be the position of my informants leads him to overlook the context in which present-day scientists and would-be observers encounter one another. Let me add a dose of twentieth-century reality.

There *is* a considerable power differential between one cultural anthropologist and the members of the knowledge engineering community—but the power in this case lies with the observed, not the observer. In choosing to investigate scientific practice in this community, I am "studying up" (Nader 1977), observing the work of people whose status (for reasons of gender, disciplinary affiliation, and access to resources) is higher than my own. The people who eventually became my informants were under no compulsion to let me into their lab in the first place and remain fully capable of throwing me out. Their power over my presence and activities is heightened by the fact that I am on their payroll: since the beginning of 1987, my informants have paid me to work with them. However, they do not throw me out, as Fleck seems to imagine they must. Instead, we have become colleagues, albeit colleagues with rather different points of view. While our divergent disciplinary orientations are sometimes a source of frustration as we struggle to work together across a paradigmatic divide, they are also a source of humor. Fleck's concern about "racist" stereotypes to the contrary, I occasionally tease knowledge engineers about being "techies"; they respond with jokes about anthropologists.

Knowledge engineers are by no means without a voice; my paper addresses received opinions which they express with confidence. Mainly faculty members and postgraduate students at major American universities, my informants can and do publish their views about all sorts of things, including what counts as legitimate scientific knowledge. While Fleck seems to find my comments unduly critical, the general perception of "soft" social science in the AI community is far more negative than my critique of their practice.

Finally, I want to address Fleck's implication (again reminiscent of colonial anthropology) that my informants cannot read and judge my work for themselves. I routinely ask the knowledge engineers in the Lab to read and comment upon what I write about them; their feedback is invariably helpful. Although he has never used it, by explicit agreement the Laboratory head has veto power over material that he sees as potentially damaging to the lab. He reads the work I submit to journals and conferences, and has patiently criticized successive versions of "Engineering Knowledge." If this paper indeed portrays him and his colleagues as "primitive savages," which is most certainly not my intent, they have not objected to it. If Fleck means to imply that these highly educated and intelligent people are incapable of noticing such a portrayal, then it is *he* who insults them, not I. What I believe instead is that the knowledge engineers understand perfectly well what Fleck does not: that different disciplinary frameworks lead people to view the same problems quite differently, and that making such differences explicit is both intellectually and (for system-builders) practically worthwhile. This is the reason I wrote "Engineering Knowledge," and it remains the rationale for my ongoing work in the Lab.

# CHAPTER SIX

# Artificial Intelligence Invents Itself: Collective Identity and Boundary Maintenance in an Emergent Scientific Discipline

This is a report from an ongoing ethnographic study of a series of artificial intelligence (AI) laboratories in the United States.[1] The researchers in the laboratories (referred to below as "the Lab") are knowledge engineers: computer scientists who specialize in developing the complex computer programs known as "expert systems." Such a system is designed to automate human decision-making first by encoding a specialized body of knowledge (known as "knowledge base") used by one or more human experts in making some particular type of decision, and second by manipulating that knowledge in order to generate specific decisions. (For further information on expert systems, see Harmon and King 1985; Hayes-Roth, Waterman, and Lenat 1983; and Johnson 1986.)

In previous papers (chs. 2, 3) I described several aspects of the cognitive and behavioral style shared by knowledge engineers at the Lab. The present paper turns outward to look at the disciplinary universe in which the knowledge engineers see themselves as operating. My approach will be twofold. First, I want to look at the collective identity that knowledge engineers construct for themselves: what do they believe themselves to be doing when they "do AI"? what kind of a field do they believe AI to be? Second, having looked at the content of the category "artificial intelligence," I want to examine its boundaries: where do its practitioners see AI as fitting in relation to other disciplines? How firm are the boundaries between AI and its disciplinary neighbors, and how are those boundaries maintained?[2]

Artificial intelligence is a particularly suitable context in which to examine collective identity and boundary maintenance among scientists. There is considerable debate within the field about just what "artificial intelligence" means, a fact that not only facilitates research on the topic but also illuminates some characteristics of the field itself.

First, the goals that AI's practitioners have set for themselves are very broad. Although there is disagreement about what the scope of the field should be, in general terms AI is concerned with the project of understanding and automating human intelligence (some practitioners leave out the word "human"). In the words of AI's founding father, John McCarthy, "The goal of [AI] is that one should be able to make computer programs that can do anything intellectual that human beings can" (quoted in Johnson 1986: 13). Although the goal of automation is not so widespread, that of understanding and modeling aspects of human intelligence is common to many disciplines, including anthropology, sociology, psychology, and philosophy. This practically ensures that the boundaries of AI will be subject to dispute.

Second, AI is a young field whose formal beginnings coincided with the development of digital computing machinery in the middle of this century. Artificial intelligence was first named and described by John McCarthy in a research proposal to the Rockefeller Foundation in the mid-1950s. The foundation funded a conference held at Dartmouth College in 1956 that focused on the question of whether machines could be made to simulate intelligence. From its very beginning, then, AI as a field has been a product of self-conscious invention. As one Lab member put it, "AI is a dream."[3] However, as psychologists know, dreams lend themselves to a wide range of interpretations.

Third, there is a great deal of money in AI at present—most of it from military sources—and the field has grown extremely fast over the past decade. Consideration of the nature and desirability of present and future applications of AI again provides considerable fuel for debate.

For various reasons, then, the meaning and appropriate scope of "artificial intelligence" are subject to ongoing negotiation, both in the literature and in day-to-day discussion in the laboratory. These processes are the subject matter of this paper.

THE SETTING AND THE FIELD RESEARCH

The data presented here derive from my field research in a series of academic laboratories, beginning in 1986. The central focus of the description is the laboratory in which I have spent the most time, referred to below as "the Lab." In addition, I draw on material from interviews and observations in a commercial AI laboratory in Silicon Valley (1987–88), on interviews with AI researchers from still other laboratories, and on texts from both the published literature and the computer bulletin boards available on the Arpanet (e.g., AIList).

The Lab is situated on the campus of a major university, and it consists of three linked sub-laboratories. All are staffed by knowledge engineers engaged in building expert systems; however, the sub-labs differ somewhat in the types of expert systems they produce. One specializes in the creation of medical expert systems, while the other two build systems related to classes of problems in other domains deemed "interesting" by the sub-laboratory heads. The sub-labs differ to some extent in the approach they take to building systems, so that the administrative divisions also reflect some degree of paradigm conflict. Altogether the Lab contains over 100 members, including faculty, research associates, graduate students, and support staff.

My field research at the Lab took place over a period of 21 months between 1986 and 1988. During that time I was a full-time participant-observer, present throughout almost every working day and sometimes in the evening as well. For 17 of those months I was on the payroll of the Laboratory itself as a full-time researcher.

CONSTRUCTIONS OF IDENTITY: ORTHODOXY AND DISSENT

Now we turn to the main theme of this paper, the problem of collective identity and boundary maintenance in AI. By "identity" I refer not to the development of an individual sense of self, but rather to the sense that practitioners of AI have of themselves as members of a category by virtue of their work. Identity in this sense is collective, and defines itself in opposition to that of other disciplinary categories perceived as different.[4]

Collective identity is created and maintained through a process of ongoing negotiation. At the Lab, this occurs in the course of the conversations, meetings, and conflicts that make up the scientists' daily work life. Statements with implications about the identity and boundaries of the field are relatively frequent, both in the Lab and in the AI literature. This paper will focus on two dimensions of such negotiation. First, Lab members negotiate about the *content* of the category "artificial intelligence"; that is, about the nature of the work that will be accepted within the field (or within the Lab) as deserving the label "AI." In this case, work is being placed and evaluated with respect to people's notions of what "artificial intelligence" means (or should mean in an ideal sense). Second, Lab members negotiate about the *boundaries* of the category "AI," that is, the point(s) at which work become "not-AI" and thus is seen by AI practitioners as belonging instead to other fields. In this case, work is being placed and evaluated not only with respect to the scientists' notions of what AI is and should be, but also with respect to their view of the proper content of other disciplines. In analyzing actual cases it is sometimes difficult to separate these two dimensions, since any particular negotiation may contain elements of both.

The sections below consider some of the terms in which people in AI define their collective identity. These terms then frame the space in relation to which the boundaries of AI are negotiated. The questions I want to address are the following: what do its practitioners think AI is, and is not, and how do they establish and maintain this boundary in the course of their everyday work life?

## The Orthodox Self-Presentation

In reporting "what Lab members think," I run the risk of appearing to stereotype. In any situation, individuals differ to some extent in what they think. This is especially true of people involved in an enterprise as broadly conceived as AI. However, Lab members (and possibly AI people in general) do hold some important assumptions about their field in common. This section points out some of these beliefs.

### Artificial Intelligence as Science

When AI is described by its founders and senior members, the word "science" is almost always used. Established AI researchers refer to their field with confidence as "the modern science of Artificial Intelligence" (Minsky 1988: 19), "the scientific field called artificial intelligence" (Feigenbaum and McCorduck 1984: 7), "the maturing science of Artificial Intelligence,"[5] and so forth. There is little doubt that the AI community's orthodox view of itself is that AI is a science. Not surprisingly, this perspective is widespread in the Lab.

One senior member of the field has commented that the identification with science "is appealing to those in AI because of the comforting and legitimate sound of the term 'science'" (Buchanan 1988). When Lab members refer to their discipline as a science, what do they mean?

### Positivist View of Science

The Lab members share a positivist view of science (ch. 3). While there is some debate within the field and within the Lab about whether AI should actually be labeled a science (see below), I am aware of no debate about what "science" itself means. The term as used by my informants denotes the use of experimentation and observation to "find regularities and assign causes and effects" (Buchanan 1988). As one informant said, science involves "using empirical techniques to deduce underlying natural laws." When they call their field a science, then, knowledge engineers portray themselves as engaged in the discovery of truth.

### Artificial Intelligence as the Science of Intelligence

Artificial intelligence defines itself as the science of intelligence. However, what is meant by "intelligence" in this context is subject to some debate within the discipline. Different "schools" in AI take a somewhat different approach to this issue.

Some AI practitioners clearly aim to illuminate the nature of human intelligence, or at least intelligence of the sort possessed by living creatures. They view electronic brains as models of biological brains whose functioning illuminates that of the living nervous system. Minsky, for example, exhorts his followers: "We must work toward building instruments to help us see what is happening in the brain!"[6]

Other researchers view intelligence as a more abstract entity that can be investigated in its own terms without reference to the brain itself or to any particular possessor of a brain. This approach is illustrated by the following definition by Shortliffe, who uses the concept of "intelligent action" without reference to the source of the intelligence involved:

> Artificial intelligence research is that part of Computer Science concerned with symbol manipulation processes that produce intelligent action. Here *intelligent action* means an act or decision that is goal-oriented, is arrived at by an understandable chain of symbolic analysis and reasoning steps, and utilizes knowledge of the world to inform and guide the reasoning [original emphasis] (Shortliffe 1986: 7).

People at the Lab take the latter approach, which is essentially pragmatic. Asked whether their expert systems are intended to model the decision-making strategy of human experts, they generally say no. They want their systems to solve problems at least as well as human experts do, they say, but do not care whether the programs use the same route to the solution that a human would take. Several commented that they hope the systems will improve upon human intelligence by finding better solutions to particular problems than people do. However, Lab members appear little interested in theoretical discussions of what "intelligence" means, or in attempts to model human cognition. In defining AI as the science of intelligence, then, I believe that Lab members place much more importance on the concept of "science" than on that of "intelligence."

### Artificial Intelligence as "Hard" Science

When senior members of the field define AI as a science, they compare it with such disciplines as physics and chemistry—fields that Minsky refers to as "successful sciences" (Minsky 1988: 322). McCarthy compares AI with genetics: "I think that this [AI] is one of the difficult sciences like genetics, and it's conceivable that it could take just as long to get to the bottom of it" (quoted in Johnson 1986: 13). As the fields chosen for comparison suggest, when AI is described as a science by Lab members or other members of the field, what they mean is what they call "hard science." They explicitly dissociate AI from so-called "soft science," to which category they assign the social sciences. This insistence on AI as "hard science" reflects the fact that the knowledge engineers universally view their work as technical in nature.

Elsewhere I have discussed the Lab members' technical orientation in relation to their cognitive and behavioral styles, calling attention to what I have called their "engineering ethos" (ch. 3). The knowledge engineers' perception of their work leads them to approach *as technical* not only tasks involving hardware and software, but also those concerned with social relations. This is illustrated by their approach to knowledge elicitation, the face-to-face interview process by which data are gathered for the knowledge base of an expert system. Observing these interviews, I noticed that even knowledge engineers with warm personalities adopted a cold interactional style when doing knowledge elicitation. When I asked such an individual why he seemed to turn off his empathy when interviewing, he replied, "It just seemed that we were doing this technical task. There wasn't *room* for empathy."

### Artificial Intelligence as Experimental Science

As we have seen, in the collective identity constructed by AI's senior practitioners, the field appears as a "hard" science. It is also portrayed as an experimental science. For example, in a report on MYCIN, one of the earliest and most influential expert systems, the authors assert, "We believe that AI is largely an experimental science in which ideas are tested in working programs" (Buchanan and Shortliffe 1984: 19). According to this view, expert systems and other complex computer programs correspond to the experimental apparatus of physics or chemistry; building and testing such systems enables scientists to prove or disprove theories in the realm of AI.

> Programs are implementations of models. Models are instantiations of theories. Theories . . . can be empirically tested by writing programs. . . . If the theory states that certain phenomina [*sic*] can be produced from a set of processing assumptions and a set of data, and a program embodying these assumptions and using such data cannot produce the phenomina [*sic*] to a level of abstraction acceptable to the theory, then the theory is disproved.[7]

Buchanan lists six steps involved in "the best experimental research" in AI. His list combines "theoretical steps" with "engineering steps" and "analytical steps," and is presented with the comment that AI researchers too often omit the last two to four steps.

> Theoretical Steps:
>     Identify the problem.
>     Design a method for solving it.
> Engineering Steps:
>     Implement the method in a computer program.
>     Demonstrate the power of the program (and thus of the method).
> Analytical Steps:
>     Analyze data collected in demonstrations.
>     Generalize the results of the analysis (Buchanan 1988).

The experiments performed in AI using computer programs are perceived as "controlled experiments":

> In calling AI an *experimental* science, we presuppose the ability to perform controlled experiments involving intelligent behavior, which are much more easily done with computer programs than with people (Buchanan 1988).

What do these experiments actually consist of? Lab members build expert systems in narrow prototype form; they are commonly referred to as "toy systems." These systems work on a small range of data, but tend to "crash" if extended outside of their limited repertoire of "training cases." As one Lab member explained,

The systems we work on around here are toys. No one's going to use them. Too expensive. Too unreliable. And they need a knowledge engineer to maintain them.

Despite the assertion cited above, then, the Lab's experimental prototypes are not "working programs" in the sense of fully implemented systems. Rather, they are designed to demonstrate that a particular approach to solving a particular problem *could* work if the builder took the time and trouble actually to implement the system.

From the standpoint of what I have called the "orthodox self-presentation" in AI, it is the limited nature of toy systems that makes them scientific; science is believed to be about ideas as opposed to implementation. The knowledge engineers contrast scientific experimentation in AI with "real-world" concerns and assign the latter to engineering:

> It's not that it's not real [the toy systems approach]. It's just a question of how much detail you go into. It's a question of engineering mindset versus a scientific mindset. I'm interested in scientific ideas. I think anything in AI these days is pretty remote from real systems.

Toy systems, then, are not intended to be practically useful; in that sense, they do not "work." Rather, they are created as simplified solutions to particular problems. Lab members see simplification as an essential strategy for their form of experimentation. Expressing impatience with people from "the humanities" who criticize AI researchers for failing to grasp the complexity of the phenomena they model, one Lab member explained the rationale for this approach:

> The scientific and engineering attitude is pragmatic. There are vast problems, but if you just simplify them they're not such a big deal. Instead of wasting n years and q careers writing papers nobody reads, just simplify a bit and solve the problem!

To sum up this section, in the three-plus decades of the field's formal existence, researchers in AI have constructed a collective identity for themselves as practitioners of a "hard" science in which complex computer programs are used to illuminate experimentally the nature of intelligence (whatever that is taken to mean). However, not everyone in AI subscribes in full to this orthodox self-presentation. Within the Lab, and within the field in general, there is some dissent. The next section considers the nature of such dissent.

## Dissenting Views

During my fieldwork, I talked with a good many individuals who took issue with aspects of the image of AI described above. All of these people are active in AI research. However, in contrast to the purveyors of the orthodox view of AI, who tend to be mainline members of the discipline, many of the dissenters seem slightly marginal in AI terms. The individuals quoted here are "marginal" in one of two ways. Some of them hold advanced degrees in other disciplines as well as AI, which may give them a different perspective from colleagues trained solely in AI. The others are graduate students, who may not yet be completely socialized into disciplinary orthodoxy. The dissenters' views may be cause and/or effect of their position in the discipline.

### Is Artificial Intelligence a Science?

Some knowledge engineers reject the notion that AI should be called a science. They do so on the basis of a number of grounds. First, some dissenters object that AI is not a separate field at all. Of these, some say that they are not sure where it belongs in the disciplinary map. This position was taken by several individuals who now work in AI but were trained in other fields.

> It's not very clear what is AI and what is not. I wonder to what extent AI is a different way of looking at problems or programming problems. [Asks rhetorically:] If you've written a program, what makes it AI?

A number of Lab members, both fully fledged researchers and graduate students, said quite seriously (in the words of one), "I don't know what AI is exactly."

In contrast, other respondents denied the scientific status of AI on the grounds that AI is really a branch of engineering, which they did not classify as a science. Speaking of knowledge engineering in particular, an AI expert from outside the Lab said:

> Expert systems is a set of programming techniques. . . . There are a few techniques and they can be useful, but that's it. Expert systems will mature into a well-understood engineered technology.

He went on to say:

> AI isn't the science of intelligence as biology is the science of living things. . . . AI is not a science. A science is dominated by using empirical techniques to

deduce underlying natural laws. An engineer [the speaker is including AI practitioners] is satisfied because something works. A scientist is satisfied because something is explained.

A Lab member commented:

> I don't know what AI is exactly, but I don't believe it's a science. It's a turf battle. AI is just software engineering.

A few informants went even further than this, denying that AI is a science not only because "it's just software engineering" but also because they objected to what they saw as exaggerated, even dishonest claims made on its behalf by some popularizers of expert systems technology. In their view such distortion is unscientific. One Lab member said of AI:

> It's a self-sustaining illusion independent of empirical bases. Statistically speaking AI and reality are independent, uncorrelated variables.

On the issue of "whether AI is really AI" (his words), another knowledge engineer expressed equally negative views. Asked to comment on a particular paradigm dispute within the discipline (see below), he exclaimed:

> It doesn't matter if cf's [certainty factors] are mathematically unsound. I think the whole programs [i.e., expert systems] are unsound!

Many of these comments assume a dichotomy between science and engineering; the logic seems to be that if AI is part of engineering, it cannot be a science. Debate on this theme has a long history in AI (ch. 3; Partridge 1987), and clearly continues.

Another set of informants expressed reluctance to call AI a science on precisely the opposite grounds—that work in AI is insufficiently related to work in other disciplines. For these people, refusing to call AI a science was an expression of their disagreement with AI's attempts to set itself apart from other fields. However, they agreed that AI could and should become a science.

*Lab member*:    AI is a science that many people say should not exist because they're just taking a messy approach to ideas that are being explored in computer science and elsewhere.

*Anthropologist*:    So would you call AI a science?

*Lab member*:    It's an alchemy. I'm trying to make it a science. Hence my paper "Towards a Science of AI". . . . AI would have become a science if there were no problem bringing in results from other disciplines. Cutting off the umbilical cords to other disciplines is really silly.

Pondering my question about the scientific status of AI, a colleague at the Lab commented:

True scientists don't think much of AI. That's because it's not precise. You can't reproduce the results. Maybe AI isn't a science and shouldn't be called a science. Maybe it's really engineering. But even in engineering you can reproduce things.

He went on to say,

I'm beginning to realize that AI is thinking about stuff that people have been thinking about for centuries—intelligence and so on. Artificial intelligence keeps reinventing the wheel.

*The Nature of Experimentation in Artificial Intelligence*

Some respondents took issue with AI's presentation of itself as an experimental science. One Lab member with a background in laboratory science was disturbed by the prevalence of toy systems in AI. He commented that AI people rarely implement their ideas by building working systems; instead, he said, they just talk about how a system would work if it *were* built. Asserting that AI is only interested in problems that haven't been solved conceptually, he charged that people in the field are not concerned with attaining working systems with real functionality. Once AI researchers know how to solve a problem in theory, he said, they couldn't care less about the actual implementation—even if the theoretical solution is "way up in the air."

In AI people get credit for talking about beautiful concepts, but they don't actually work. But then when someone comes along and actually implements the idea, he doesn't get any credit for it because it's already been talked about.

In support of these comments, this researcher cited his own unhappy experience. At the Lab, he had worked for many months to implement in a working system a set of concepts that a project colleague had developed. However, a manuscript describing this achievement had been rejected for publication on the grounds that the *idea* had already been published. This researcher's bitter assessment of the values of AI practitioners was supported when I later spoke with the colleague whose ideas he had implemented. The colleague said of this researcher, "He's just a C programmer." [C is a computer language.] It was in part this experience that led the researcher to conclude that "true scientists don't think much of AI."

## Collective Identity in Artificial Intelligence

While disagreeing about whether AI should be called a science, Lab members actually share a number of underlying assumptions. The most important of these is the concept of science that lies at the core of their collective identity as practitioners of AI. Together with a body of associated ideas, this central concept frames the territory within which they struggle to define themselves professionally. Note that both orthodox "AI as science" people and dissenters retain their respect for "hard science" and for scientific experimentation, as well as sharing a positivist understanding of what science is. They do not question whether science is a good thing or whether scientific work actually conforms to the positivist model. Rather, what Lab members debate is whether AI *qualifies* as a science. I suggest, therefore, that their contradictory statements should be seen not as negations of each other, but rather as part of an ongoing dialogue through which the identity and the boundaries of AI are negotiated.

AN EXTERNAL VIEW

Thus far I have taken a relativistic approach in reporting on the views of the knowledge engineers. Now I would like to step back for a minute and draw on my observational experience in order to comment on two aspects of the professional identity that the knowledge engineers have constructed for themselves. In making these comments I make no claim to be more correct than my informants; it is rather the case that my perspective as an outside observer and a social scientist leads me to perceive certain matters differently than they.

First, when social scientists look at AI, they often form an impression that conflicts with a central tenet of both AI's orthodox self-presentation and the dissident views discussed above. Anthropologists and qualitative sociologists familiar with the knowledge engineering process[8] have commented on its resemblance to the data-gathering and analytical procedures of their own disciplines (Collins 1987b: 345–6; Forsythe and Buchanan 1989; Woolgar 1985: 558). Viewed from the social science side of the boundary, it appears that there is considerable overlap between these disciplines: whereas the practitioners of AI see themselves as doing "hard" science, observers on the other side of the disciplinary boundary see parts of AI at least as indisputably "soft." Whether or not the knowledge engineers think of it in this way—and in my experience they do not—knowledge engineering appears to an anthropologist to be centrally concerned with problems of order and translation.

The knowledge engineers in the Lab have very little interest in qualitative social science or indeed in any approach that strikes them as "soft." For example, when the Lab asked me to discuss interview procedures with student knowledge engineers, I began with material about human social interaction; special attention was given to such factors as gender and cultural background. Most of the students seemed to find this material irrelevant. They told me that they were interested in learning "techniques rather than ideas" —a distinction that an anthropologist finds difficult to make. The few knowledge engineers I have encountered with any interest in qualitative social science are people who happen to have a personal relationship with an anthropologist or social psychologist. In these cases, interpersonal factors have apparently succeeded in overcoming the knowledge engineers' professional conviction that "soft" social science is irrelevant to their field.

My second comment concerns an apparent contradiction between the knowledge engineers' self-presentation and the nature of their work. Whether or not they see themselves as "scientists" or "engineers," Lab members take a pragmatic approach to their enterprise. When this enterprise is challenged from outside—for example, from the social sciences or from other "schools" of AI (e.g., connectionist research)—their answer is invariably, "We don't need to worry about that—what we're doing works!" Such claims abound in AI. Calling AI "this critically important technology," for example, Feigenbaum informs us, "With AI, the role of the computer in our lives changes from something useful to something essential" (1985: v). Ironically, though, what the knowledge engineers are doing doesn't work. By their own account what they are building are "toy systems," "experiments" that are not designed to work in the sense of having any real-world utility. Indeed, it appears that to build a system that really *does* work is to court low prestige in academic AI and to run the risk of being labeled "just a programmer."

I suggest that both the phenomena described here are consequences of the nature of the collective identity that AI has chosen to construct for itself, in combination with the assumptions they bring to that undertaking. Because they view "hard" science as antithetical to "soft" science, the AI establishment's defense of its members as "hard" scientists leads them to reject input from the social sciences. Because they define themselves as scientists, and view science as unconcerned with implementation—the putative realm of engineering—they have relatively little interest in building systems with real functionality.

## HOW IDENTITY IS USED IN BOUNDARY STRUGGLES

As we have seen, science and its attributes serve to frame the collective identity that AI constructs for itself. These same ideas and assumptions are used as legitimating concepts in the course of boundary disputes, both within AI and between AI and other disciplines. In such disputes, the scientific virtues are used as weapons: typically, each party attempts to establish its own claim to science and its attributes while ruling the opposition out of the category "scientific" and if possible out of the category "AI" as well.

Not every characteristic of either AI's disciplinary boundary or the space within that boundary is subject to negotiation and dispute. For example, despite the view from outside the discipline (see above), there appears to be no internal dissent to the notion that the work of AI is exclusively technical. Within the field, this belief appears to have the status of tacit knowledge (Polanyi 1965)—information so obvious to AI practitioners that it is rarely articulated.

Similarly, there seems to be little or no negotiation about the exact location of AI's boundary with the neighboring social sciences, although this boundary is heavily defended from within. The knowledge engineers' concern appears to be to deny the boundary's existence rather than to locate it.

However, AI practitioners do engage in claims and counter-claims concerning other aspects of their disciplinary identity and its boundaries. This section presents an example illustrative of this process. The example itself is very simple, and yet as we shall see it relates to several important disputes in AI.

### An Illustrative Example

Speaking of a major research project carried on under his direction, a senior scientist at the Lab says occasionally in a rather critical tone, "That's not AI" or "They're not doing AI." The speaker is a well-known AI researcher referring to work undertaken by his own doctoral students and by research associates paid by his laboratory. He is a principal investigator on the project and is listed as an author on project publications. So what does it mean when he says of this research, "That's not AI"?

## Explication

The professor is saying a number of things at once. His comment expresses his position on a series of interrelated disputes within the Lab involving technical questions, the proper content of AI as a discipline, and the location and desirable strength of the boundaries of the field. Some of these issues are outlined below.

### Issue 1: Technical Dispute

The first issue is an ongoing dispute about the relative merits of different techniques for encoding uncertainty in the knowledge base of an expert system. When he says of a particular expert system "That's not AI," the professor is making a statement about his position in this dispute. Some background information will be necessary to clarify this.

The university where the Lab is located is well known in AI as the place where some of the earliest expert systems were developed. The knowledge bases of these systems consisted of a large set of rules which contained information about uncertainty in the form of heuristics (qualitative "rules of thumb") and so-called certainty factors (known in the Lab as cf's). These certainty factors were subjective estimates of uncertainty translated into quantitative form (from $-1$ to $+1$) for computer processing. According to their creators, cf's are not probabilities and do not rest on any formal mathematical underpinning; rather, they constitute a technique developed through trial and error that was adopted because "it worked." Having been used in a major early expert system, this approach to encoding uncertainty became standard at the Lab for many years.[9] Its originators came to see the use of this type of method as *definitive* of AI.

Recently, however, a different approach to building expert systems has come into use in one of the sub-labs, borrowed from the field of decision science. This method uses a quantitative technique for encoding uncertainty, replacing certainty factors and qualitative rules of thumb with explicit, mathematically formal statements of probability which are manipulated within the expert system according to the rules of Bayesian statistics. Rather than using certainty factors, practitioners of this newer approach attach to each piece of information in the knowledge base a precise numerical weight on a scale from 1 to 100. Along with other information, these weights are "extracted" from the expert in the course of knowledge elicitation (ch. 3).[10]

Lab members disagree about the relative merits of certainty factors (plus heuristics) and Bayesian probabilities for use in expert systems. The senior researcher in our example was involved in the development of some early rule-based expert systems and is committed to their use. However, some of his current students and junior colleagues have become converted to the use of Bayesian systems, and the project mentioned in our example is developing a Bayesian system. Thus, when the professor says of a particular project "That's not AI," on one level he is differing from them about a technical matter, their choice of a particular method of encoding uncertainty in the expert system being developed in the project. However, there are other issues involved here as well.

### Issue 2: Science and Disciplinary Boundaries

Researchers in favor of using the Bayesian approach say that because it incorporates a formal statistical technique, their method is more exact than the less formal approach based on heuristics and certainty factors. Therefore, they claim, the Bayesian method is more scientific. Those in favor of using certainty factors counter that such a statistical approach may be exact, but it isn't AI. They also point out that it is very difficult to get an expert to explain his personal expertise in terms of precise statistical probabilities; even if he does produce such data, it's not clear what they mean. Non-Bayesians tend to criticize this approach as offering only the illusion of science.

In this dispute, then, one side claims "science" for itself, implicitly labeling its opponents "unscientific." The other side makes a counter-claim about the boundaries of the discipline, defining its own approach as "AI" while trying to exclude from that field the work of its opponents. It also questions the scientific status of the Bayesian approach. Beneath the technical issues lie some differences in *values* concerning not only the meaning but also the relative merit of "science" and "artificial intelligence."

### Issue 3: Allegiance to Science vs. Allegiance to Artificial Intelligence

The example highlights a conflict of allegiance facing the knowledge engineers. At issue is their accountability to AI as a discipline, on the one hand, versus their accountability to science as a global endeavor, on the other.

As we have seen, the Bayesian approach incorporates theory and techniques from other disciplines, including decision science and statistics. From the standpoint of its proponents, borrowing from other disciplines is a perfectly sensible thing to do. Indeed, they point out, science depends upon this process of building on older foundations without regard for disciplinary boundaries. As one Lab member explained, "I'm very interested in seeing science as a common activity, showing links between AI and other disciplines." Another commented, "You see a problem and solve it as best you can. There is no special need to use _____ [a famous rule-based system built in the Lab]." The first allegiance of these knowledge engineers is to science as a global activity; they see the use of AI techniques for their own sake as parochial. Furthermore, they point out, the apparent determination to invent everything themselves rather than drawing on other disciplines condemns AI researchers to unnecessary work. As one Lab member said, "AI keeps reinventing the wheel."

However, there is a counter-position held by other AI researchers. As they point out, undertaking research in AI means to do work in that field, not in statistics or decision science. Since AI is a pioneering field, it is important to use and improve the techniques developed in AI. Part of the reason for their lack of enthusiasm about some interdisciplinary research may also be a certain feeling of disciplinary insecurity. Because AI lacks the historical tradition of such sciences as physics, some of its practitioners worry about the status of their field and debate how to gain acceptance for it as a valid discipline in its own right. This insecurity may contribute to their reluctance to acknowledge the relationship between AI and neighboring fields. I have the impression that people taking this position may see the discipline itself as threatened by the readiness of some researchers to ignore its boundaries and search for solutions in other fields. To return to our example, then, the phrase "that's not AI" can be seen as an expression of alarm concerning such boundary-crossing as well as an attempt to shore up the boundaries by sounding the alarm.

CONCLUSION

As we have seen, AI has constructed for itself a collective identity framed in terms of science and its attributes. These same ideas and assumptions are used as legitimating concepts in the course of boundary disputes, both within AI and between AI and other disciplines. In such disputes, scientific virtues are used as weapons: typically, each party attempts to establish its own claim to science and its attributes while ruling the opposition out of the category "scientific" and if possible out of the category "AI" as well.

The case of AI is of interest to the social study of science for several reasons. First, it allows us to explore the process by which an emergent scientific discipline struggles to define its own identity and to set boundaries between itself and neighboring disciplines. Second, it illustrates some of the problems faced by such a discipline. For example, the knowledge engineers wrestle with the tension between trying to establish AI as an independent discipline, on the one hand, and either borrowing from other disciplines on occasion or having to duplicate their work. And third, it illustrates the compelling nature of science as a concept, a concept so powerful to the founders of AI that the discipline is inventing itself in its image.

# CHAPTER SEVEN

# New Bottles, Old Wine: Hidden Cultural Assumptions in a Computerized Explanation System for Migraine Sufferers

Computers have now been in use in medical settings for several decades.[1] Since the early 1970s, computer systems incorporating artificial intelligence have been developed with the goal of providing decision support for clinicians and (more recently) patients.[2] Both builders and users of such systems tend to think of them simply as technical tools or problem-solving aids, assuming them to be value-free. However, observation of the system-building process reveals that this is not the case: the reasoning embedded in such systems reflects cultural values and disciplinary assumptions, including assumptions about the everyday world of medicine. The processes by which such values and expectations come to be inscribed in new computerized technologies are largely unexamined.[3]

This paper draws upon my eight years of full-time participant-observation in the world of intelligent systems. I focused upon software design in medical informatics, a rapidly growing field at the intersection of computer science and medicine.[4] Presenting material from a project to build a computerized patient education system for migraine sufferers, the paper addresses two themes. First, how do values and expectations come to be embedded in technology? As I will show, software developers do not necessarily intend to do this and, indeed, are often not even aware that they do it. This raises the problem of agency. Second, what are the implications of this state of affairs? I argue that the embedding of tacit values in biomedical technologies raises issues of importance for both practitioners and consumers of medical care. These issues include questions of knowledge and power between doctors and patients. Some of the assumptions inscribed in knowledge-based systems are contested in the world of medicine and/or in the wider society. Designed into software, however, they become invisible to the user and thus unlikely to receive much scrutiny (chs. 2, 3).

These points are grounded below in specific examples from the system-building project. First, however, I present some background on anthropological studies of computing and on the migraine project.

BACKGROUND

## Locating Technology

As Suchman (1994) has noted, technology is always located. Although the designers who build such systems may think of the artifacts they produce as transcending social particulars, tools are inevitably used in specific practice settings. As I will show, tools are also created in specific practice settings.

Location in Suchman's sense is a matter of place and practice. In his analysis of the computerized medical decision support system known as ACORN, Berg elaborates the notion of location, addressing "localization" in space, scope, and rationale (Berg 1997: ch. 4). In the present paper, I argue that technology is located in another sense as well, in terms of the origin and nature of the ideas it embodies. The attempt to unpack intelligent systems conceptually, from a cultural and disciplinary standpoint, is a central theme of my research in artificial intelligence and medical informatics.

Designers of intelligent systems tend to portray them as "objective, neutral agent[s]" (Crevier 1993: 362), thus positioning (what they see as) computerized reason outside the unpredictable social and cultural contingencies of everyday life. Anthropologists have increasingly contested this construction, however, locating such technologies instead in the social and cultural world of their designers. Ethnographic observers have documented the embedding in knowledge-based systems of a wide range of beliefs and expectations carried over from the everyday world (ch. 1; Graves and Nyce 1992; Kaplan 1987; Lundsgaarde, Fischer, and Steele 1981; Nyce and Lowgren 1995; Nyce and Timpka 1993; Suchman 1987, 1990). For example, such systems have been shown to represent beliefs about the relation between plans and human action (Suchman 1987), expectations concerning the nature of work practice in particular settings (Suchman 1992), theories about individualism and education (Nyce and Bader 1993), and tacit assumptions about the nature of knowledge (ch. 3) and work (ch. 2).

These anthropological analyses of the system-building process and of the software thereby produced show consistently that intelligent computer systems are cultural objects as well as technical ones. Because they are often taken for granted, the assumptions embodied in system design can be invisible to those who hold them. Since such beliefs are not necessarily shared by end-users, however, their representation in a system may contribute to problems of comprehension or acceptance when the software is installed in real-world settings (see ch. 2; Suchman 1987).

The assertion that designers build aspects of their own worldview into their systems in unacknowledged and uncontrolled ways has found little resonance in computer science and medical informatics. Most designers apparently do not believe that they build cultural values and assumptions into their systems. Indeed, they do not always recognize that they *hold* some of the values and assumptions that I and other observers have pointed out. While it is not unusual for anthropologists' accounts of others to differ from the others' accounts of themselves, this difference in perspectives is intriguing because it raises the problem of agency. Ideas do not embed themselves in technology, nor do I entertain the determinist notion of humans as "cultural dopes" (Garfinkel 1967: 68, quoted in Suchman 1990: 307). If identifiable cultural and social expectations *are* routinely represented in intelligent systems, just how do they come to be there?

In addressing this question, I present examples from a three-year project to build a natural language patient education system for migraine sufferers (Buchanan, Moore, Forsythe, Carenini, Ohlsson, and Banks 1995).[5] Design involves decisions made daily throughout the long process of system-building. Such choices reveal many things decision-makers take for granted. In the case of the migraine project, these involved not only abstract cultural and disciplinary beliefs held by various members of the design team, but also assumptions about such things as what counts as "medical knowledge," power relations between doctors and patients, the relative importance of nurses, the reasons for (what physicians call) patient "non-compliance," and other characteristics of the everyday world of medicine.

The investigation reported here is highly reflexive. As an anthropologist studying a scientific community engaged in formulating knowledge descriptions, I offer my own descriptions of their knowledge. In addition, as explained below, I carried out ethnographic fieldwork not only on a system-building project, but for it. Based on that fieldwork, I also describe something of the knowledge of migraine sufferers. My attempt to describe and contrast different sets of assumptions inevitably reveals some of my own beliefs as well. In the text below, I use my own reactions and experiences to help throw my informants' assumptions into relief.

## The Migraine Project

In 1991, a university-based research team received funding to support a three-year, interdisciplinary project to design and build a computerized patient education system for people with migraine. The system was intended to empower migraine sufferers by providing them with information about their condition and its treatment. In contrast to conventional design procedures in medical informatics, this project included ethnography; the latter was used not only to document project meetings but also to provide input to system design. Fieldwork included observation of 78 doctor-patient visits in neurology, informal interviews with numerous physicians and patients, and extended formal interviews with 13 migraine sufferers (Forsythe 1995). Formal interviews and most of the doctor-patient encounters were audiotaped. A detailed content analysis was carried out on the 600-page transcript of 18 of the doctor-patient visits.[6]

A prototype system was built and subjected to formative evaluation with migraine patients. Intended to be used by both patients and doctors (or other health care providers), the system consisted of two linked components: a history-taking module and an explanation module. The development team intended the system to be used as described in the following scenario.

> A new headache patient comes into the doctor's waiting room and is invited to sit down at the computer to use the system. First, the history-taking module presents an automated questionnaire, which takes a detailed initial history of the patient's headaches. Based on the user's responses, the system prints out a written summary for the neurologist to use when seeing the patient. Before subsequent visits, the system takes a shorter update history, again producing a written summary for the physician. Following each encounter with the doctor, the explanation module of the system is available for patients to use to pursue questions of interest to them. Since the history-taker sends information to the explanation module, which also receives up-to-date information about the patient's diagnosis and medications from the physician, the system is able to provide on-screen explanatory material that is tailored to each individual patient. This material contains information about the patient's condition and current medications, offering further explanation as desired. In addition, it includes some general (i.e., non-tailored) information about the experience and treatment of migraine on topics seldom addressed explicitly by doctors. Several levels of explanation on each topic are offered, activated when the user clicks with the computer's mouse on words and phrases of interest in

each text screen. When the patient is finished using the system, the computer prints out a record of the explanatory material presented that day for the patient to take home.[7]

Three factors contributed to our choice of migraine as the focus of the explanation system to be built by the project. First, migraine is very common. This chronic condition inflicts severe and unpredictable pain on approximately 20 percent of the population (Lane, McLellan, and Baggoley 1989). Three-quarters of migraine sufferers are women (Saper, Silberstein, Gordon, and Hamel 1993: 93). Second, although this condition causes great discomfort (Good 1992), it is almost never fatal—a quality that attracted the research team on ethical grounds. While the goal of the system was to help migraine sufferers, the team was reassured by the knowledge that failure to help patients would be unlikely to cause them lasting harm.

And third, the fact that the diagnosis and treatment of migraine depend upon effective verbal communication between physician and patient made it an attractive domain for a system-building project. Few physical signs or laboratory tests differentiate this condition from other sorts of headache. Instead, diagnosis depends primarily on a thorough history of symptoms; treatment efficacy is evaluated on the basis of what the patient reports. Since information that humans articulate can also be requested and provided in text on a computer screen, the research team expected migraine to be a suitable domain for the provision of explanatory material by means of a computer.

## Locating Myself in Relation to the Migraine Project

This paper is part of an extended field study in the anthropology of science and technology, focusing upon the relationship among the values and assumptions that practitioners bring to their work, the practice that constitutes that work, and the tools they construct in the course of their work. I take an interpretive approach (Geertz 1973, 1983), attempting to understand what events mean to the people involved. From 1986 to 1994, I was a full-time participant-observer in five software development laboratories in the United States. Four of these were located in academic settings; one was in an industrial setting. The unusual length of this fieldwork reflects the complexity of the technological and social processes under investigation; systems typically are produced collaboratively and take several years to develop.

The migraine project took place during the last years of my fieldwork. In the beginning of the project, at least, I was a full participant. I wrote substantial portions of the funded proposal, which explicitly proposed the use of ethnography to support system design. Paid by the project as a co-investigator, I took an active role in group meetings and coordinated the ethnographic fieldwork and analysis.

As the project progressed, however, I found it increasingly difficult to reconcile my roles as both participant and observer. The paradigmatic differences between informaticians and anthropologists that I had documented in my previous work (chs. 2, 3) took on practical as well as epistemological significance as we attempted to find ways to reconcile relativist understandings of ethnographic data with the positivist expectations and procedures of normal system-building. As the project developed (steps outlined below), I became less of a participant in and more an observer of the system-building effort. Despite our shared initial intent to undertake an innovative design effort, despite the rich ethnographic data on migraine that we collected and analyzed for the project, and despite some anthropological contribution to the explanatory content and overall direction of the prototype system (Forsythe 1995), the migraine system that was actually built reflected much less ethnographic input than we had originally envisioned. Some of the reasons for this outcome will become apparent in the following sections.

## DESIGNING VALUES AND EXPECTATIONS INTO AN INTELLIGENT SYSTEM

The design team included people from computer science, cognitive psychology, medicine, and anthropology. In the course of the three-year funded project, these people met in various combinations for dozens of project meetings. During these meetings, and during informal discussions between them, team members made decisions that affected the design of the system. The design decisions described below were the outcome of negotiations to which individual team members sometimes brought divergent points of view. In order to protect their privacy, I refer to team members collectively and omit details of how particular decisions were made.

Design decisions reflect different levels of intentionality. Some are made explicitly. Others occur as a sort of side effect of other, explicit decisions, while still others can be said to occur by default. (It may be inappropriate in the latter case to use the word "decision.") To convey a sense of these three possibilities, I will give examples of each.

1. An explicit design decision: "hanging" explanatory text on the patient summary. The migraine system was designed to engage in an explanatory dialogue tailored to the specific needs of the user. In order to initiate the dialogue, the system-builders needed to present users with something to ask questions about. For this purpose, they chose to use the so-called patient summary—a two- to three-page text presented on the computer screen that details the neurologist's recommendations during his or her most recent visit with the migraine patient. This text averages about ten paragraphs in length and is adapted to each patient around a basic topic structure. A sample text begins as follows:

> Today you were seen by Dr. _____, who diagnosed you as suffering from migraine. The most common symptom of migraine is a moderate to severe headache. Migraine patients also frequently experience visual symptoms, nausea, sensitivity to light, sensitivity to noise and confusion. Your head may feel tender and sore when you have a migraine headache. Much of the pain in a migraine headache is thought to be due to the stretching of blood vessels in the scalp and the head. Your symptoms included flashes, light-spots, double-vision, blurred-vision, photo phobia, and painful-eye-movements, which are all consistent with typical cases of migraine.[8]

Patient summaries go on to mention that migraine is hereditary, that migraine attacks may be frightening but are rarely life-threatening, and that they are likely to get better with age (a comment offered only to women who are premenopausal because of the frequent connection between migraine and the menstrual cycle). They describe migraine triggers and address the treatment and possible side effects of medications prescribed for the particular patient using the system. The designers considered the decision to "hang" the system's explanatory texts on the patient summary to be straightforward. However, this choice had a significant tacit consequence for users that the system-builders either did not notice at the time or simply took for granted.

2. Tacit consequence of an explicit design decision: excluding explanatory material from the system. Because explanations are displayed when the user clicks on words or phrases in the patient summary, the prototype system cannot explain anything that does not fit into the scope of this text. The system design thus excludes patient questions on topics that were not addressed by doctors during patient visits. This prevents the system from answering most of the questions we picked up from migraine sufferers during fieldwork, which

were unanswered in the first place because they involved topics not generally addressed by doctors during patient visits. Even though the design team never actively decided to ignore patient questions that lay outside the scope of what doctors prefer to talk about in the office, in effect they did just that.

3. A default design decision. A third type of design "decision" is not a conscious decision at all, but rather an unplanned reflection of the designers' worldview. Like everyone else, software designers make assumptions about the everyday world; these may affect their work practice. For example, an unconsidered omission by the migraine system designers prevents the history-taker from collecting potentially important information about the user's possible experience of domestic violence. The question below is from the section of the automated questionnaire intended to establish the user's headache history:

> Did anything happen to you at about the same time you started having this kind of headache?
> _____ accident
> _____ illness
> _____ started or stopped some drug or medication
> _____ other
> _____ don't know
> _____ not applicable

If the user checks "accident," a pop-up window appears on the screen and offers three further options:

> _____ head injury
> _____ injury other than a head injury
> _____ car accident

This question sequence categorizes physical injury under "accident." The questionnaire thus does not allow for the possibility of headaches caused by *intentional* violence, a significant omission given that 75 percent of migraine sufferers are women (Saper, Silberstein, Gordon, and Hamel 1993: 93). Physical trauma is a relatively common cause of migraine (Weiss, Stern, and Goldberg 1991), and domestic assault is a form of trauma to which women are particularly vulnerable. On the basis of observations and transcript analysis, the project ethnographers had noted that several of the women in our study appeared to be victims of domestic violence; this point had been mentioned repeatedly at research team meetings. Nevertheless, because of a particular, perhaps gender-biased view of the world, the men who wrote the above question for the history-taker did not make the connection and overlooked a possible cause of post-traumatic migraine that mainly affects women.[9]

I have illustrated the fact that system-builders' tacit assumptions can affect the design of an intelligent system in a variety of ways, reflecting different degrees of intentionality. The next section describes how particular assumptions were inscribed in the prototype migraine system at different stages of the development process.

## ASSUMPTIONS EXPRESSED IN THE DESIGN OF THE MIGRAINE SYSTEM

Some design decisions affected the user interfaces to the history-taking and explanation modules (i.e., what appeared on the screen). Others affected the way the system worked and what it could address, but remained backstage from the user's standpoint. Decisions of both types were influenced by designers' cultural and disciplinary assumptions.

The sections below provide examples of both types of decision. I organize them sequentially, in order of the major stages of system-building: (1) assembling the project team, (2) problem formulation, (3) knowledge acquisition, (4) writing the code to build the system, and (5) evaluation. Obviously, assumptions made by designers in one stage of system construction are likely to be made in other stages as well. For reasons of convenience, I discuss particular assumptions in the context of design decisions that reflect them especially clearly.

### Stage I: Choosing the Project Team

The stated goal of the migraine project was to develop a patient education system for the benefit of migraine sufferers. The research team assembled for this project was large, containing half a dozen faculty members, two programmers, a research assistant, and about six graduate students.

Two aspects of the composition and interaction of the team are of note. First, the team contained two physicians but no nurses. In view of the fact that nurses often have a great deal of contact with patients and consider patient education to be one of their most important jobs, their absence from the project is noteworthy. It reflects the characteristic muting of nurses' voices in medical informatics in relation to those of physicians.[10]

Second, the voice of migraine sufferers was muted as well on the project, although for somewhat different reasons. Although four non-physician members of the research team (including two senior members) actually suffered from migraine, they spoke in meetings only in their professional roles; they never spoke in their private personae as migraine sufferers. This was especially striking because in private interviews, they had eloquently described to me the pain and fear of their migraine attacks, and the failure of biomedicine to provide them with significant relief—a story heard over and over again in the course of the study. Yet for three years, they remained silent about these experiences at project meetings, allowing the physicians (none of whom had migraine) to speak for patients. Although these migraine sufferers' private stories diverged from the project physicians' accounts of what migraine patients know and want to know, they never publicly contradicted these physicians. I see their silence as reflecting the power differential between doctors and patients in the world of medicine. Their choice (in public, at least) to privilege "expert" medical knowledge over their own experiential knowledge may also reflect the stigmatization of migraine to which several of our interview respondents referred.

Insofar as it affected the work that produced the migraine system, this disparity of voices between doctors and nurses, and between medical experts and lay people, is inscribed in the system design. What migraine patients know and say in private about their condition is present in the system only as it was represented on their behalf by physicians and anthropologists. And whatever nurses might have had to say about migraine and its treatment is completely absent from the system.

## Stage II: Problem Formulation

Intelligent systems are intended to solve problems. Problem formulation, the initial design stage, involves deciding what problem a prospective system should address. This decision in turn influences the type of system to be built.

The project team made a series of assumptions that led to the definition of the problem that the migraine system was to address. These assumptions were not all explicit; indeed, as beliefs taken for granted in medical informatics, many remained completely tacit. Below I recapitulate the basic argument made by the project team during problem formulation, considering several of the assumptions on which this argument rests.

*Basic Argument*

1. Physicians know a great deal about migraine.

2. Migraine sufferers need this knowledge in order to manage their condition better. In the language of medical informatics, migraine sufferers have unmet information needs.

3. These information needs contribute to (what physicians see as) the problem of poor patient compliance: if patients knew more about migraine, their compliance would improve.

4. Improved patient compliance would promote successful treatment of their condition, which in turn would empower them.

5. Physicians do not have time to provide patients with lengthy explanations and are likely in future to have even less time for explanation.

6. The problem to be solved, then, is migraine patients' insufficient access to medical information, which in turn is caused by the time shortage of physicians. Since information needs can be met by delivering more and better information, and since intelligent systems are well suited for information delivery, there is a clear need for an intelligent system to provide patients with explanatory material about migraine.

*Assumptions*

To some, this argument and its conclusion may not seem to rest upon assumptions at all, but upon obvious truths. As the foundational assumptions of medical informatics, these "truths" are so thoroughly taken for granted that they are invisible to people within the field. But as the fieldwork with migraine sufferers made clear (Forsythe 1995), the steps in this argument can be viewed from other points of view. Below I recapitulate the assumptions enumerated above, pointing out some issues of perspective.

1. The project team assumed that knowledge about migraine means biomedical knowledge, that is, formal, general information of the sort found in medical textbooks (Forsythe, Buchanan, Osheroff, and Miller 1992).

2. Because the project team interpreted "knowledge about migraine" to mean what doctors know, they believed that migraine sufferers who are not physicians lack knowledge about migraine. As I began interviewing migraine sufferers in private, it became clear that this assumption is wrong. People with migraine tend to know a great deal about the condition and about some of the drugs used to treat it. They may have different knowledge than physi-

cians. For example, people with migraine have experiential knowledge of what happens to them during migraine attacks, which they often exchange with fellow sufferers. In addition, they may have medical knowledge. Some of our informants read medical literature about their condition and were extremely well informed. In relation to physicians, then, migraine sufferers may have *alternative* knowledge but certainly do not *lack* knowledge about migraine.

3. The migraine team assumed that the information needed by migraine sufferers was biomedical information. They expected patients to want physiological information about migraine and about the side effects of drugs used to treat it. In other words, the research team simply assumed that what patients wanted to know about migraine is what neurologists want to explain. In actuality, however, migraine sufferers expressed a desire to know about a broad range of topics involving migraine, beginning with the apparently universal secret fear, "Do I have a stroke or a brain tumor?" (Forsythe 1995).[11] Much of what they said they wanted to know about their condition was informal and/or specific knowledge (Forsythe, Buchanan, Osheroff, and Miller 1992) rather than textbook material. Of particular importance to people living with migraine was the problem of translating formal medical knowledge about migraine and its treatment into information that they could apply in their own lives, a factor that seems related to patient compliance (Hunt, Jordan, Irwin, and Browner 1989).

4. The migraine team assumed that lack of time prevents physicians from explaining more to patients. However, our observation of patient visits suggested that time is not the main factor constraining explanation to patients. In fact, a great many questions are asked and answered during patient visits, but almost all of them are asked by the doctor and answered by the patient. This finding is consistent with the literature on doctor-patient communication (Frankel 1989; Wallen, Waitzkin, and Stoeckle 1979, quoted in West 1984: 108). We found that neurologists provide relatively little explanatory material and that patients are given little chance to request it. We also found that when patients attempt to bring up concerns that neurologists do not see as strictly medical, physicians often appear not to "hear" them or attempt to pass the matter off as a joke. Such patient concerns include veiled references to death (presumably prompted by the secret fear mentioned above [Forsythe 1995]) and questions about how they can carry on normal life and work in the face of unpredictable disability. Clearly, migraine patients *do* have unmet infor-

mation needs, but they are not necessarily due to a lack of physicians' time. On the basis of our observations, I would attribute such information needs as well to the power of physicians to control doctor-patient discourse and thus to avoid topics they may not be prepared to address.

In the problem formulation stage, the migraine team defined a problem they saw as technical in nature. Given this view of the problem, they proposed a technical solution: development of a computer system to deliver to migraine patients the information they were assumed to need.[12] As I have tried to show, the team's construction of the problem took for granted a series of assumptions and expectations about the medical world. These included the privileging of biomedical knowledge over the knowledge of patients and a tendency to overlook the power of doctors to avoid patients' questions. Not only were the research team's assumptions and expectations embodied in their problem formulation; as I show below, they were also built into the system.

## Stage III: Knowledge Acquisition

The proposal to use ethnography in support of system design was innovative. I was convinced that concepts and methods from anthropology could make a useful contribution to software design and evaluation (Forsythe and Buchanan 1989, 1991, 1992). Although a handful of social scientists have applied ethnographic and survey methods in medical informatics since the 1970s (Anderson and Jay 1987; Kaplan 1983; Kaplan and Duchon 1988; Lundsgaarde, Fischer, and Steele 1981; Nyce and Timpka 1993), social scientific contributions to design are still viewed as experimental by most people in medical computing. Perhaps because writing code is seen as the "real work" of software development (see ch. 2), ethnographic research tends to be subordinated to the conventions of "normal" software design. In the present project, for example, senior physicians and computer scientists were unwilling to have fieldwork with migraine sufferers begin before the writing of code for the migraine system. Instead, it was decided that fieldwork and system-building should run in parallel.

The anthropologists began systematic fieldwork at the start of the funded project. We observed interactions between patients and neurologists, and we conducted private interviews with migraine sufferers and physicians. At the same time, the system-builders began to think about how to represent the knowledge that they expected the fieldworkers to present to them. However, tensions arose over the issue of timing. Accustomed to a "rapid prototyp-ing" model of software production, the designers wanted to start building the system long before the anthropologists felt ready to generalize from the early field data. In order to have something to code, the designers began conventional knowledge acquisition in parallel with the ethnography. Their intention was to build results of the ethnography into the system as they be-came available.

Elsewhere I have written about what conventional knowledge acquisition entails (chs. 2, 3; Forsythe and Buchanan 1989). In the migraine project, it involved debriefing a single neurologist (designated as "the expert") about migraine drugs, treatment strategies, drug side effects, etc., and then incor-porating his conscious models into the knowledge base as "knowledge about migraine."

The plan to combine the results of this knowledge acquisition process with the results of the ethnographic investigation reflects the system design-ers' assumption that knowledge is neutral. In computer science and related fields, knowledge is generally viewed in positivist terms. It is assumed that one can understand and evaluate it in decontextualized fashion without at-tention to the identity or position of the knower (ch. 3). In medical infor-matics, knowledge is conventionally described in terms of transfer and flow. "Information needs" are seen as "out there," stable (at least in the short term), inherently ordered, characteristic of and shared by groups or cate-gories of people, and knowable by others. Thus, one task expected of the anthropologists on the migraine project was to "find" the information needs of migraine patients and to report them (in a prioritized list) to the system-builders. Seen from this reifying perspective, knowledge should be additive. It made sense to the designers to begin building the system's knowledge base by representing material supplied by the physician-expert, with the intent of incorporating the ethnographic findings later on.

In contrast, anthropologists see knowledge as inherently contextual (Geertz 1983). To consider knowledge "needs," "transfer," or "flow" with-out addressing the matter of who wants, knows, or shares this knowledge is (for an anthropologist) to delete an essential part of what it means to know. Furthermore, because all human beings are positioned in a social order, their knowledge is seen as positioned as well. To an anthropologist, knowledge always incorporates a perspective (Rosaldo 1993). Given this view, knowl-edge is neither neutral nor necessarily additive.

It turned out to be difficult to combine the results of conventional knowledge acquisition with the insights from fieldwork. The material obtained by the conventional method embodied a neurologist's point of view. It privileged the knowledge and categories of formal medicine and incorporated the assumptions and expectations characteristic of medical informatics. In contrast, the ethnographic findings treated physicians' and patient's perspectives on migraine as different but equally valid. While the designers were willing in principle to encode such material in the system, in practice it just did not seem to fit. The ethnographic material was inconsistent with design elements to which they had committed in the early stages of conventional knowledge acquisition with the physician-expert. Later on, material based on the ethnography was difficult to incorporate into the system because it did not take for granted the centrality of medical events (e.g., the doctor-patient visit) or a physician's point of view.

## Stage IV: Building the System

In addition to the general epistemological and disciplinary assumptions discussed thus far, the migraine system also embodied more specific assumptions and expectations of the research team. Below I illustrate specific assumptions that were built into the history-taking and explanation modules.

### Design of the History-Taking Module

The history-taker is an automated questionnaire that inquires about the user's headache and medication history. Each patient's responses are compiled to create a printed summary for the physician. The responses are also passed to the explanation module, which makes use of them to generate explanatory text tailored to the gender, age, symptoms, medications, migraine triggers, and other attributes of each individual user (Buchanan, Moore, Forsythe, Carenini, Ohlsson, and Banks 1995).

The migraine team included several social scientists who were experienced in constructing and piloting questionnaires. However, the job of developing the history-taker was given to a computer programmer, who approached the assignment as a system-building task. Rather than first developing and refining a set of questions, as a social scientist would have, the programmer built version after version of a computer system that *generated* questions—a much more difficult undertaking. The questionnaire produced by each version of the system was criticized by fellow team members, after which yet another version of the entire module was slowly and carefully built.

Eventually, perplexed at the seeming irrationality of constructing successive versions in code instead of in simple text (which would have been much faster), I asked the computer scientist in charge why the social scientists had not simply been asked to construct a questionnaire, pilot it, and then give it to the programmer to code. The response highlighted different disciplinary assumptions concerning the nature of the work in question. From my standpoint, the automated history-taker was a questionnaire. I saw its construction as a social science task that happened to require some programming to represent the final product. From the computer scientists' standpoint, in contrast, constructing the history-taker was a technical task because the material was to be represented in code. To them, it was a coding job that happened to involve a questionnaire.

This distinction expresses a significant difference in perspective. To computer scientists, the "real work" of constructing the history-taker was writing the code, that is, producing the computer program that generates what the user sees on the screen and that processes information supplied by the user. This stance reflects the centrality of coding work in computer science (see ch. 2). For computer scientists, "getting the words right"—their understanding of the social science contribution to both questionnaire and system design—was merely "frosting on the cake." To an anthropologist, in contrast, constructing a good questionnaire raises epistemological issues about the categories into which human experience is divided. From this viewpoint, resolving such issues was an important part of the "real work" involved in constructing the history-taker. This contrast in perspectives reveals conflicting assumptions about the relative importance of technical work and epistemological work (or, alternatively, about which part of the work should be seen as technical.)

The design of the history-taker also reflected a second kind of assumption, the belief that migraine sufferers categorize their headaches as a physician would. The wording of certain items in the dynamic questionnaire generated for each user privileged medical categories and a physician's perspective. For example, at the beginning of a history-taking session, users are asked: "How many types of headache do you have? Answer the questions about the type that brings you to the doctor today." This question reflects the assumption that headache patients classify their headaches according to the same "types" that neurologists use. Therefore, one of the types is expected to be migraine. However, this assumption was not borne out by our field data, which showed that headache sufferers may categorize their experience quite differently from neurologists. For example, a patient diagnosed as suffering from both migraine and tension headache, or from two different types of migraine, may understand herself to be suffering from one fluctuating or unpredictable "type" of headache. In this case, her responses to the history-taker would "lump" information about what a neurologist would see as two different types of headache.

### Design of the Explanation Module

As with the history-taker, the interface design for the explanation module reflected the assumed centrality of medical perspectives and events. As noted above, all explanatory material in the prototype system is "hung" on a summary of the doctor's recommendations during the patient's latest visit. The prototype system is restricted to explaining items that can be worked into the context of this text. This is a severe constraint. Our observation showed that neurologists rarely bring up issues outside the formally medical (e.g., lifestyle questions) and tend not to respond to patients' attempts to bring up such issues (e.g., concerns about whether particularly severe attacks may be fatal). Based on the fieldwork, I compiled a list of about 200 queries to which migraine sufferers wanted to know the answers. The restriction of the system's explanatory frame to the patient summary made it impossible for the system to address most of these questions. Instead, members of the project team made up questions for the system to answer. In effect, then, they worked around the ethnographic data in order to revert to conventional design procedures.

The system reflects in several ways the assumption that patients are passive and physicians are active and powerful. For example, as illustrated above, for more than a year the prototype patient summary began, "You were just seen by Dr. _____, who diagnosed you as having migraine." This language frames the user as object in relation to the physician. Late in the project, it was finally changed to "You just saw Dr. _____, who diagnosed you as having migraine," thus removing from the explanation module one small symbolic representation of the power differential between physicians and patients.

However, other potentially more disempowering aspects of the system design remain unchanged. As is conventional among computer scientists who design natural language systems, the developers saw the purpose of the explanatory dialogue produced by the explanation module as *persuading* the user to believe certain things. This stance is reflected in their description of the system's text planning architecture, excerpted below:

> The explanation planning process begins when a *communicative goal* (e.g., "make the hearer believe that the diagnosis is migraine," "make the hearer know about the side effects of Inderal") is posted to the *text planner*. A communicative goal represents the effect(s) that the explanation is intended to have on the patient's knowledge or goals [Buchanan, Moore, Forsythe, Carenini, Ohlsson, and Banks 1995: 132] [emphasis in original].

The system selectively presents information to headache patients in order to try to persuade them to believe certain things deemed appropriate by the designers. For example, the initial paragraph of the patient summary (see above) defines migraine *in the general case* for a given user by listing the specific symptoms selected by that user while taking the headache questionnaire. Thus, if Mrs. Jones experiences flashes, light spots, double vision, blurred vision, photophobia, and painful eye movements in connection with her headaches, the patient summary subsequently constructed for her by the explanation module will list these as typical symptoms of migraine. Symptoms of migraine that Mrs. Jones does not select on the questionnaire do not appear in the general description of the condition shown to her. This design feature is intended to "make [Mrs. Jones] believe that the diagnosis is migraine."

In short, the system has been designed to persuade patients that the physician's diagnosis of their headaches is correct. This aspect of the design takes for granted two major assumptions. First, it assumes that the physician's diagnosis *is* in fact correct, although no test exists to verify a diagnosis of migraine. Second, the suppression of typical migraine symptoms not experienced by a given patient from the general description of migraine implies that it is more important to persuade patients to believe their physician's diagnosis than it is to present them with information that might serve as a basis for doubting that diagnosis. Although such assumptions were never explicitly raised at project meetings, their incorporation into the system design seems more likely to empower physicians than patients.

Finally, the explanation system embodies a physician's perspective not only in what it explains to patients but also in the way in which concepts are explained. Despite our data about what migraine patients want to know, the explanatory material actually offered by the prototype system largely reflects the physicians' assumptions about what patients need to know. It also reflects physicians' notions about what constitutes proper explanation. Examination of some of the explanatory text produced by the system suggests that such assumptions can be wildly inappropriate on both counts.

The three pieces of text below were all drafted by a physician for the explanation module and encoded in the prototype system. The first text piece contains essentially no explanation at all; the second offers an explanatory image likely to disturb any user; and the third consists of textbook-type language so inaccessible that it offers little illumination.

1. Material intended to address the experience of headache:

> Well, everyone has a tender or sore head at some time. If you bump your head on a wall you would expect it to be sore. On the other hand, if it is sore as part of your migraine, then it may be part of the migraine symptomatology.

2. Material intended to address the question of whether an individual's migraine triggers will always cause a migraine attack:

> Triggers in the case of migraine can be likened to the trigger on a gun. When pulling the trigger on a gun there will sometimes be misfires when the gun does not go off. This also seems to be the case in migraine. A trigger is therefore a physical or mental action that OFTEN causes the onset of headache, but not necessarily always.

3. Material intended to explain the causes of migraine:

> The precise causes of recurring headache as in migraine are not known. There is a belief that the pain originates from structures of the brain, specifically the nerve systems which travel to and from the spinal cord. It is believed that there is a disturbance of transmission system. This means that there is a problem in the way the nerve impulses travel to and from the brain. No specific personality type has been implicated. It is not thought to be a neurosis or a psychosomatic disorder. The conventional view of the cause of classic migraine, dating from the early observations of Wolff and his colleagues, has been that vascular narrowing accounts for the neurological symptoms and the dilation of the vessels for the headache and tenderness. The pulsatile character of the headache seems to indicate a vascular factor. More recent theories place greater emphasis on the role of sensitized nerve endings in the blood vessels, which release a chemical substance called substance P; this causes the vasoconstriction or narrowing and therefore a regional reduction in blood flow. Another hypothesis

favors an initial disturbance of the hypothalamus and limbic cortex; the latter are two centers in the brain. None of these hypotheses explains the periodicity of migraine.

## Stage V: Evaluation of the System

Researchers in both medical informatics and anthropology devote considerable attention to questions about information and knowledge. However, as we have noted, they understand these concepts rather differently. During the evaluation of the prototype migraine system at the end of the three-year project, the questions that the computer scientists and anthropologists wished to ask of users of the system reflected these different views of knowledge. The specialists in medical informatics focused upon the quantity and utility of the information offered by the system. One of their concerns was to demonstrate that the system offered patients more information than their doctors had in the past. This goal is reflected in the following question contributed by a computer scientist to the interview schedule for the evaluation of the prototype system:

> Did the program ask for less or more information than doctors you have talked to about your headaches?

In contrast, my questions focused upon the perceived meaning and appropriateness of the information offered to the user. As the interview schedule developed, I contributed questions such as the following:

> Did the information presented make sense to you? [If not] What didn't make sense?
>
> Was anything presented that seemed confusing or inappropriate to you?

Such divergent questions about the system reflect different views of knowledge.

DISCUSSION

Koenig has described the tendency for expensive new technologies to "diffuse into widespread clinical practice before evidence is available about their actual usefulness" (Koenig 1988: 467), a phenomenon that reflects what Fuchs called the "technologic imperative" in medicine (Fuchs 1968, 1974). Medical computing does not fit this pattern. Although medical information systems are being developed at a rapid rate, it is common for technically sound systems to be rejected by their intended users and not adopted into clinical practice (Anderson and Aydin 1994: 6). In medical informatics, this phenomenon is known as "the problem of user acceptance" or "end-user failure." As these labels imply, when computer systems are not accepted into clinical practice, system developers tend to blame the users (ch. 1).

My research on system design in medical informatics reveals another factor relevant to the so-called problem of user acceptance: the fact that systems embody perspectives that may not be meaningful to or appropriate for their intended users (Forsythe 1995). As I have tried to show in the case of the migraine system, the dozens of design decisions made by different members of the project team embodied some assumptions and expectations characteristic of medical informatics in particular and of biomedicine in general. The composition and interaction of the project team reflected the muting in American medicine of the voices of nurses and patients. The formulation of the problem that the system is intended to address, and the choice of an intelligent system as a solution to this problem, reflected foundational assumptions of medical informatics. The organization of the work of system-building reflected characteristic assumptions about the importance of "technical" in relation to epistemological work. And the restriction of the system's explanation capability mainly to facts about physiology, drugs, and drug side effects reflects the bias in American medicine toward formal, biomedical knowledge—despite the ethnographic data gathered for the project that showed migraine sufferers to have pressing concerns of a less formally medical nature (e.g., how to live with a condition that can cause unpredictable and incapacitating pain).

These assumptions will not startle anyone familiar with the everyday world of American medicine. However, it may be startling that such assumptions should be built into a "neutral, objective" piece of technology—especially one intended to empower patients. Whatever the good intentions of the builders (and I do not believe they set out to embed these assumptions in the system), the result is a piece of technology that is anything but neutral.

In a domain in which a careful observer can discern several valid points of view, the migraine system embodies only one: that of a neurologist. The content of the knowledge base and the language and categories generated by the user interface all reflect a neurologist's approach to the doctor-patient encounter and a neurologist's view of what counts as relevant medical knowledge. These biases are nowhere pointed out to users of the migraine system—not because the designers have consciously decided not to do so (to my knowledge, they never considered it), but presumably because they do not see either themselves or the system as biased. This situation raises important questions about what end-users—in this case patients—have a right to know about technology used in clinical care.

As the migraine system illustrates, software may embody values and assumptions that users might wish to question—if they were aware of them. For example, I am troubled by the fact (noted above) that the designers of the migraine system intentionally but covertly try to persuade users that their diagnosis of migraine is correct.

Unfortunately, medical diagnoses are *not* always correct. It may be that the user actually has a brain tumor instead of migraine or that (like the first patient to use our system experimentally in a headache clinic) she has both migraine and a brain tumor. By omitting from the description of migraine those symptoms the user does not experience, the system withholds information that might conceivably help an incorrectly diagnosed patient to realize that the physician has made a mistake. Similarly, the system fails to inform users that it has been designed to make them believe their diagnosis. Indeed, the introductory screen states that "This system has been designed to help you understand your condition and suggested treatment better," implying that the system is neutral. These omissions pose ethical problems.

In these and other instances, use of the system may actually increase the power differential between physicians and their patients, a situation that is even more likely in the future if members of the research team carry out their plan to expand the system. The designers intend to adapt the migraine system to individual neurologists by encoding in its knowledge base each doctor's personal preferences in medication and treatment. While one might assume such preferences to be "strictly medical," in fact some of them seem distinctly cultural. For example, one physician we observed consistently recommended one particular migraine drug to male patients and another to females. When queried about this, he said that the medication he suggests to men is his true drug of choice for migraine. But because the drug can also cause weight gain, he does not recommend it to his female patients. Believing that women either should not or would not wish to gain weight, he makes a choice on their behalf that they might prefer to make for themselves.

The designers intend to replicate such preferences in personalized versions of the system's knowledge base, justifying this plan as the only way to induce physicians to put the system in their offices. Biases in the material presented will not be pointed out to users. For example, medications that particular physicians prefer not to prescribe, or not to prescribe for particular classes of patients, will simply be deleted from the list of possible items about which users can obtain information. This, too, poses ethical problems. Furthermore, while the designers believe that physicians need to be induced to use this new technology, patients are not seen as requiring inducement to use the system. The designers seem to take for granted that patients can be made to use it by virtue of their reliance on physicians for pain relief. This pragmatic assumption reflects—and seems likely to reinforce—the power imbalance between doctors and patients in the social world of medicine.

This paper was inspired by a question of agency: how do cultural assumptions come to be embedded in complex computer programs even when system designers do not intend this? The answer I offer treats cultural and disciplinary assumptions as interpretive resources. It attributes agency neither to a reified notion of culture nor to the technology itself, but solely to the human actors. At the same time, it acknowledges that human acts do not always bring about the intended consequences.[13]

This study bridges the concerns of two newly converging research traditions within anthropology and sociology (Casper and Berg 1995; Star 1995): the study of medicine and the study of science and technology. The idea that biomedicine is characterized by hidden (and not-so-hidden) cultural assumptions is well known to medical anthropologists (e.g., Gordon 1988; Kirmayer 1988). Equally familiar are the assumptions about power and knowledge that I have attributed to neurologists and shown to have been replicated in the migraine system (e.g., Lindenbaum and Lock 1993). That the practice of science invites *cultural* as well as social analysis is still rather new within science and technology studies, however (Hess and Layne 1992). Similarly, the extent to which contested cultural assumptions are routinely inscribed in supposedly neutral technologies is becoming familiar within the anthropology of science and technology, but may not yet be so well known to medical anthropologists.

WILL THE SYSTEM HELP MIGRAINE PATIENTS?

It is worth considering whether use of this new biomedical technology is likely to help migraine sufferers. I have argued that many of the expectations of medical practice that were used to motivate development of this system in the first place are represented in its design. In a sense, then, the system itself replicates these conditions: it addresses patients as passive, determines (through its menu-based user interface) what questions the user may ask, offers explanation on the same narrow range of topics neurologists do, and avoids the sort of awkward "non-medical" questions that we observed doctors themselves avoiding in face-to-face interaction.

Although the system is intended to be used by both patients and physicians, its definition as a *patient* education system incorporates the assumption that patients can learn from physicians but not vice versa. The system presents to patients aspects of physicians' knowledge about migraines, but does not explain to physicians anything about the knowledge or experience of migraine sufferers—although we learned much about the latter during the fieldwork that could be incorporated into such a system to help educate neurologists about the experience of migraine.

Most importantly, the system does not allow patients to speak for themselves. Even in a condition diagnosed through patient history, the system compels users to fit their diverse personal stories (Good 1992; Good, Brodwin, Good, and Kleinman 1992) into neurological categories. As Berg notes in the case of ACORN, such disciplining of real-world complexity to the formalisms embedded in a computer system is required to enable the tool to work (Berg 1997: ch. 3). The designers of the migraine system could at least have created special boxes in the interface for users to type free text into the system on designated topics, to be read later by the physician. However, they chose not provide this feature.

One might wonder, then, if use of the system in a clinical setting would ameliorate or exacerbate the problems it is intended to solve. At this point it is too soon to tell, since the system is still in prototype form and has only been used experimentally in a neurology clinic and in the development laboratory. Shortly before the end of my fieldwork, however, I took part in the first round of evaluations of the system. Interviewing three volunteers who had spent several hours talking with a neurologist and using the history-taking and explanation modules, I asked each one (among other things), "How did you feel about having a computer give you this type of information? Would you rather get such information from a human being or a computer?"

Despite my own expectation that users would not—or perhaps should not—like the system, these three people did like it. They justified their views with precisely the reasoning given in the migraine project proposal. One user commented that doctors do not have time to answer questions but that the computer never got impatient; another noted that while she sometimes felt stupid asking questions of the doctor, she felt free to question the computer. When the system made errors (e.g., "forgetting" what a user had just told it about factors that triggered her migraines; or referring in error to the tyramine-free food list that "your doctor just gave you" when he had not), these users forgave it.

But brief experiment is not the same thing as normal use, and three is much too small a number from which to generalize about users' reactions to the prototype system. The system would have to be more fully developed and many more people would have to use it before conclusions could validly be drawn about any effects of its use. Nevertheless, this initial step in evaluation does serve as a reminder that not only designers but also anthropologists bring assumptions to their work: end-users may see a piece of technology differently than a critical observer.

CONCLUSION

Where should we locate the migraine system? Most of the project team would probably place it in some neutral scientific space, far from the disorderly world of the everyday. While they are aware that they have embedded some assumptions in the system, they consider these to be minimal, necessary for system-building, and appropriate to the domain.

In contrast, I locate the system in the disciplinary and cultural worlds of its creators. I am struck by the extent to which they have built assumptions from their respective worlds into the system. In decisions about work practice and system design, they have expressed a wide range of tacit and sometimes explicit expectations concerning themselves as doctors and patients, as specialists in "hard," "technical" work, as knowers and dispensers (but not recipients) of medical information, and as people in a gendered world that systematically overlooks the skills and experiences of nurses and victims of domestic violence. The migraine system is in no way a neutral technical object. Rather, it is a kind of collective self-portrait of its designers, revealing little about its intended users but much about those who built it.

In closing, I return to the notion of the technological imperative in medicine. The tools of medical computing have not been adopted into clinical settings as readily as the treatment technologies described by Koenig (1988). While technology *adoption* in medical informatics has been slower than expected, however, technology *production* in this field is escalating rapidly.

The decision to build the migraine system certainly reflects a technological imperative. Practitioners in medical informatics take for granted the benefits of automation, including computerizing doctor-patient communication that might otherwise take place face-to-face. In medical informatics, intelligent systems technology is treated as a solution in search of a problem. "Research" in this field means building a system; "problem formulation" means finding a real-world justification for the system one wishes to build. Left aside here are important questions about the broader costs and benefits of this approach for defining and sharing medical knowledge. Whose assumptions and whose point of view are inscribed in the design of technical systems? Who will benefit from adoption of a given system, and who stands to lose? As the case of the migraine project demonstrates, the answers to these questions are not simple nor are the questions themselves necessarily even apparent to users. If designers do not ask such questions, and users are not always in a position to do so, who will monitor the hidden cultural assumptions built into computerized tools for medicine?

# CHAPTER EIGHT

# Ethics and Politics of Studying Up in Technoscience

The past two decades have seen enormous growth in the type of research that Laura Nader has called "studying up" (Nader 1972, 1977, 1980).[1] This change is both cause and consequence of two other trends in anthropological research. First, the concern of the late 1960s and 1970s to "bring anthropology back home" (Berreman 1972; Cole 1977; Wolf 1972) has been heeded. Large numbers of American anthropologists now carry out field research in Western industrial societies, including the United States. Of these, a significant proportion choose to study up. For example, research in my own field, the rapidly expanding anthropology of science and technology, almost always involves studying up in the United States. Second, the feminist anthropological practice of using research as a means of cultural critique (Morgen 1989) has been taken into the disciplinary mainstream (Marcus and Fischer 1986). It is now common for anthropologists to study powerful institutions and agencies within the United States with an agenda that includes some amount of explicit critique.

These developments in the discipline as a whole are reflected in my own research career. Twenty-five years ago, I began doing fieldwork in small communities from minority cultures in remote rural areas of Scotland, then studied urban Germans, and now find myself very much "back home," studying the cultural nature of scientific truth—widely seen as our own most authoritative knowledge.

In this paper I draw upon my own experience to reflect upon the changing nature of anthropological work. I argue that not only is studying and critiquing the powerful itself a considerable departure from previous practice in our discipline, but the locations from which many of us do this work both reflect and create important changes in the nature and potential consequences of anthropological fieldwork.

## DISRUPTING THE TRADITIONAL FIELDWORK NARRATIVE

What one might call the "traditional fieldwork narrative" in cultural anthropology goes something like this. An anthropologist based in academia receives a grant to carry out a field project. She journeys to "the field," which is far from home, possibly picturesque, probably small and rural, and very likely inhabited by people who bear little relation to her home society, class, profession, or employing institution. If they read, they may not read English; if they are aware of the anthropologist's conclusions about their way of life, their opinions concerning the quality and utility of her analysis are unlikely to influence her future career. While in "the field," the anthropologist's lack of expertise in local work skills and perhaps in the local language limit the degree of real participation open to her. She remains more or less a visitor, the very "otherness" of the setting implying that sooner or later she will go home. In short, the "field" and "the informants" who there reside belong to a distant, parallel universe whose inhabitants have no power over—and possibly little knowledge of—the funders, journals, faculty committees, and potential employers who inhabit the world of "home."

The kind of research that concerns me here disrupts this tale in almost every possible way. The relocation of fieldwork and fieldworkers to powerful institutions in this society has major implications for the conditions under which field research takes place and the kinds of relationships that develop between anthropologists and their informants. Not only are the basic premises of the traditional narrative unlikely to apply under these new conditions (for example, going "away" to the field may mean crossing the campus to a different building—or simply going to work at one's company), but some important role distinctions assumed in this narrative have a tendency to disappear.

My paper undertakes two tasks. First, drawing examples from my own ten years of research on computer scientists and doctors, I describe some of the ways in which studying up in the United States disrupts this traditional fieldwork story. While few individual aspects of this divergence will be surprising—many of them follow from the very definitions of "studying up" and "working in the United States"—in combination they amount to a major change in the nature of ethnographic work and the conditions under which it is accomplished. Second, I argue that these changes have significant consequences for both the fieldworker and those she studies. One such consequence is a blurring of distinctions in terms of which fieldwork has traditionally been defined. This alters the relationship between studier and studied, increasing their vulnerability to each other and raising some troubling ethical and political concerns.

## COMPARING THE OLD AND NEW FIELDWORK STORIES

### Old Story

I will begin by elaborating upon the basic themes of the traditional fieldwork story.

1. Fieldwork takes place "away" from the fieldworker's normal milieu, in a location that is geographically, politically, economically, socially, and culturally "elsewhere."

2. The informants' social world is unconnected with that of the anthropologist—they live in separate societies or separate classes/regions within the same society.

3. The informants are relatively powerless. While they may have a lot to say over whether and how she does fieldwork in their community, they have no power over the way the anthropologist represents them. Indeed, they may not even know how they are represented in her work. Their reaction to her construction of them has no bearing on the anthropologist's future ability to obtain jobs or research grants or to publish her material about them.

4. Professionally, the fieldworker is based in academia (probably in anthropology) and paid from a source in her own professional world. If actually living in the society in which she does the field research, she is based in an institution (e.g., colonial administration) different from the institutions in terms of which her informants' lives are structured. In either case, the anthropologist leaves her informants' community when the research is done to return to her own home society/institutions.

5. Traditional fieldwork is temporally bounded—the fieldworker remains in the field for months or years and then goes home.

6. The informants do work quite different in nature from that of the anthropologist. They may be farmers, fishermen, market women, whatever—traditional ethnographic fieldwork has rarely taken place among people whose primary work skills are lecturing, reading, writing, and publishing academic papers.

7. Lacking local work skills, possibly language skills, and the intention to

stay for the long term, the fieldworker is rarely a genuine participant in the practice she has come to observe. She remains largely a visitor, tolerated or indulged according to local circumstance. Sooner or later she goes away, back to the parallel universe of her own "real life" and career.

*New Story*

Contrast the traditional fieldwork story with the way the same themes play out when an American anthropologist studies up in the United States. I will refer to this as the "new" fieldwork narrative.

1. Fieldwork takes place among people who may be from a similar social, cultural, and class background to the anthropologist. Field sites are often geographically and culturally close to home. In my own field, for example, the anthropology of science and technology, fieldwork may take place in a building across the campus of one's own university or in a local research institute, hospital, or corporation. In a complete merging of "home" and "field," moreover, growing numbers of anthropologists carry out field research in and on institutions in which they are employed. For example, Xerox Corporation, NYNEX, General Electric, and Apple Computer have anthropologists on staff whose work includes carrying out in-house ethnographic work. In my own case, I was for a decade a paid researcher in a series of soft money labs involved in software production. Much of my time there was spent studying my own workplace.

2. In this new set of circumstances, the social worlds of fieldworker and informants may overlap considerably. This has the effect of collapsing roles that remain separate in the traditional narrative: informants may also be faculty colleagues, fellow employees, or indeed one's own employer.

3. This new state of affairs changes the power relations between fieldworkers and informants. In contrast to the traditional narrative, informants are not necessarily powerless in relation to the fieldworker; on the contrary, they may have considerable power over her. That power may continue for years after the fieldwork ends. In my own case, some of my key informants for the past decade have been the computer scientists and physicians who hired me and paid my salary. While I wrote or contributed heavily to several of the grants that supported me, I was not named as principal investigator on any of them—another of the political realities familiar to anthropologists working in/on scientific settings.

In addition to this shift, the issue of representational power also plays out differently in this new narrative. Far from being unaware of how I represent their work in print, my informants are highly interested in this question. Intelligent, highly trained people, many of them read what I write about them. Sometimes they contest it. Whereas fieldworkers in the traditional narrative may never encounter their informants' reactions to the way the anthropologist has represented them, in the new narrative the anthropologist can hardly avoid such reactions. Corporations routinely require fieldworkers to sign non-disclosure agreements; they generally also want to vet written work before it can be presented or submitted for publication. While I have never had to sign such an agreement in non-corporate settings, I find it advisable to show my paper drafts to key informants in order to get their feedback and to allow them to object to anything they might find potentially damaging. (Fortunately, few objections have arisen, but I think it would be folly not to check for that possibility.)

4. Like other American anthropologists, those who study up are increasingly located outside of tenure-track jobs in academia. Within universities, many are supported on soft money and/or in other departments; outside academia, anthropologists are finding positions in a range of agencies and corporations. This means that we who study up are increasingly paid from sources outside our own discipline; some of us are paid by the people we study.

Under these circumstances, fieldworkers investigate and critique elite institutions from a position of little or no job security—a vulnerable stance from which to challenge the powerful in one's own society. It is one thing to write critically about events halfway round the world, or for a tenured professor to publish a critique of local power structures. It is quite another for an anthropologist in a corporation or on soft money to call into question the practices of those who employ her and who may be in a position to affect her future ability to make a living. Where home and field are contiguous or even identical, there is no "elsewhere" for the fieldworker to return to.

5. Fieldwork according to this new narrative may not be temporally bounded as strictly as more traditional fieldwork. Indeed, it may have no endpoint at all. Anthropologists who carry out research in/on the institutions in which they work do not necessarily go "away" when the research is finished. For them, "home again" may mean back to their own office elsewhere in the same institution—or it may mean remaining in the very same site.

6. In this new type of research, anthropologists find themselves studying

people whose work and work skills are quite similar to their own. Many of my informants in science and technology are graduate students and people with Ph.D.'s whose daily work strongly resembles my own: we both use computers, do email, read journals, and write papers. Since medical informatics has intellectual concerns in common with cultural and medical anthropology, there is a good deal of overlap in what we read and write papers about. It is precisely such overlap in interests and work skills that makes it possible for anthropologists to locate themselves for long periods of time in laboratories and corporate settings and to produce knowledgeable critique of their practice.

7. Studying up in the United States offers the possibility for at least some anthropologists to be much fuller participants in events in the field site than is possible for many fieldworkers under more traditional circumstances. This possibility is promoted by fieldworkers' presumed possession of excellent language skills, knowledge of and membership in the wider society, academic skills (useful in some settings, at least), and the fact that the fieldworker is not necessarily constrained to go home again after a relatively short period of time.

PRACTICAL CONSEQUENCES OF THE NEW NARRATIVE:
ETHICAL AND POLITICAL DILEMMAS

I have outlined important changes in the nature of field research and of the conditions under which such work is carried out. As I pointed out, major role distinctions in the traditional story may blur or break down altogether in the new one, so that informants, funders, colleagues, employers, grant reviewers, and job referees sometimes turn out to be the same individuals. Where they are not the same, they may be members of the same professional communities—in my own case, the small world of medical informatics. Similarly, the meaning of "participant-observer" may be quite different in the new narrative, because fieldworkers observe social processes in which they are genuine and possibly paid participants.

This blurring of roles and boundaries offers both benefits and costs to anthropology, its practitioners, and the people we work with. On the positive side, relocating and redefining fieldworkers and informants in relation to each other and changing the nature of the "field" and "fieldwork" offer the possibility of deeper understanding of complex social and technical processes. This in turn provides a more solid basis for critique and—to the extent that the anthropologist is also attempting to work for her informants—greater utility to them as well.

At the same time, ethnography under the changed conditions I have laid out is bound to render fieldworker and informants more vulnerable to each other. Not only does the changed fieldwork context create new kinds of vulnerability, but the risks to both anthropologist and informants may extend far beyond the fieldwork itself.

Finally, studying up under the conditions of the new narrative can create a host of personal and professional dilemmas for the anthropologist as conflicting loyalties pull her in opposite directions and the collapsed roles of participant, observer, critic, employee, and colleague collide with one another. I will illustrate this with four examples. I could cite many more.

## Informants Read and React to the Way We Represent Them

Anthropologists who study far-away people who do not read are not likely to be faced with their reactions to the way they have been represented. Those who work with literate people in other societies sometimes publish abridged versions of their reports in local languages for their informants' consumption (e.g., Laurence Wylie's edited French version of *Village in the Vaucluse*).[2] At the other extreme, those of us who write about well-educated people in the United States can be sure that our informants will be able to read everything we publish. We can also be sure that they will not agree with everything we write.

Anthropologists take for granted that our accounts of people's lives are not necessarily identical with what those people would write about themselves. This is especially likely if one's accounts question their practice. However, this relativist assumption is not widely shared in the broader society: unless our informants are relativists and/or people of considerable tolerance, they may not make this assumption. I work with people who are largely positivists; they tend to believe that a point of view is either right or wrong and that the difference is a matter of evidence. (Anthropological evidence, however, is often dismissed as "anecdotal.") People with whom I have worked in medical informatics have generally been able to accept what I write as simply my perspective and to believe that it is at least intended to be helpful. However, others in that field (particularly people I don't know well) sometimes see my writing as simply wrong; in some cases they react to it with hostility. This can be awkward politically, since some of these individuals have been asked to comment upon my grant proposals, journal manuscripts, and applications for jobs and promotion.

Much concern has been devoted to the privilege accorded the anthropological voice and the difficulty of letting informants' voices be heard. Anthropologists who critique powerful people tend to encounter the opposite problem. Our informants *have* voices and generally have no difficulty being heard. This is of course especially true of scientists and doctors. In contrast, it is often the anthropologist—frequently less powerful than her informants—who may have trouble being heard. (I sometimes wish for a bit of that epistemological privilege as I try to persuade computer scientists and doctors to treat social and cultural meanings as more than "frosting on the cake.")[3]

Anthropologists who study up in their own society need to be aware of the following facts of life:

1. If you publish things about powerful people that they do not agree with, they will not necessarily like it.

2. Unless they are people of great generosity—and there certainly are such people—they may not wish you to continue to write more of the same.

3. This may affect your career.

4. It is especially likely to affect your career if you are (a) untenured or not based in a university; and (b) dependent upon the people you critiqued (or people like them) for employment, promotion, or research funding.

No one will be surprised by these facts of life. As they imply, however, anthropologists who study up in this country under the conditions of the new narrative are likely to be faced with some awkward trade-offs. In my own experience, it may not be possible to avoid at least some costs.

## *Should One Compete with One's Informants?*

Where role distinctions collapse, fieldworkers may find that their various loyalties and obligations conflict in confusing and ethically troubling ways. As a participant-observer for several years, each in a series of scientific laboratories, I sometimes found it difficult to know how to balance my roles as fieldworker and lab researcher. One practical issue was the question of competition with my fellow lab members, who were both colleagues and informants.

Anthropologists have traditionally felt an obligation to protect our informants' interests, or at least not to harm their interests through our work.

As a participant-observer in Scotland and Germany, I tried to help my informants to achieve their own goals. On request, I taught people to drive, baby-sat, played the organ in church, mucked out barns, corrected people's English, did translations, and so on. Such activities never seemed ethically problematic and never brought my informants' interests into serious conflict with my own.

When studying laboratories that also employed me, however, the situation has been very different. One of the main goals of scientists and graduate students in laboratory settings is access to limited resources; these include money, promotion, space, and the attention of people senior to oneself. As fieldworker, I would wish to help my informants to achieve such goals, or at least not to impede them. But as a fellow lab member, I sometimes found myself in direct competition with them. Students and researchers assigned to carrels in loud, busy rooms wanted their own offices; I wanted an office, too. Lab members wanted the lab head to read and comment upon their papers; I wanted his attention, too, for my own proposals and papers. And when I discovered that I was being paid two-thirds of what a male scientist ten years my junior was making, I wanted a raise.

So what to do? On the one hand, where resources are tight, people who don't compete may find themselves without them. I needed resources to do the work for which I was paid. On the other hand, overtly to compete with one's informants carries the risk of jeopardizing the fieldwork. Are people likely to volunteer information about their work and personal lives that they fear might be used against them? Furthermore, informants are actors as well as objects of the anthropological gaze. A fieldworker may try to be a friend to all, but what is one's ethical obligation in relation to informants who start competing with you? In one lab, a senior researcher started attacking me at lab meetings. Would I have been justified in fighting back? Would it have been ethically acceptable to fight back using information I knew from interviewing him or others? Could I have done this and continued to define myself as a field researcher in that situation? I found this situation very difficult. When the participant and observer roles conflict in this way, the traditional fieldwork narrative offers little guidance.

## Who Owns Your Data?

A third concern brings up related issues of competition and power. Who owns the data you collect with funding from your informants or from funding sources in their world? What if your informants want to use these data in their own publications? What if they want to use data you collected in ways that you feel to be ethically or intellectually problematic? This question has arisen in my own career and has arisen as well for several colleagues who do similar research. It arises in part as a consequence of the overlap between our work skills and those of our informants in science and technology studies, and often turns out to be difficult to resolve.

My informants these days are largely scientists and physicians who, among other things, write and publish papers. They are always on the lookout for data. In several work settings, my informants realized that a fieldworker who collected data about them could also collect data about others. Thus, I became a collaborator in projects in which my role included producing data about the "information needs" of doctors and patients to support the design of intelligent systems for medical settings. When one joins a collaborative project, one presumably agrees to share data within certain parameters (and I heartily recommend that these be defined explicitly and in advance). In two of these labs, however, an issue arose that brought my anthropological assumptions about data-sharing into conflict with those held by my informant-colleagues in other disciplines.

Anthropologists see observational data as the interpretive construction of the observer and, thus, view data that we collect as our own intellectual property. But in the positivist world of medical informatics, observational research is viewed as trivial: the straightforward collection of what is "out there."[4] One physician described me in my observer role as "a walking tape recorder." However, he saw lots of potential uses for the data I produced, and without my permission he passed out to his medical fellows field transcripts I had produced for a project in which they were not involved. This created a dilemma for me. As fieldworker in his laboratory, I wanted to be pleasant and useful. Obviously, my field data provided just such utility: by enabling his fellows to avoid the "trivial" but burdensome necessity of collecting empirical data, my transcripts enabled them to produce quick publications.

On the other hand, in my participant role, I was competing with those fellows. Having put in the time to collect and interpret the data, I felt that it should not be given away without my permission. This situation turned into a major struggle between two laboratory heads: my own lab head, with whom I had a mutually satisfactory agreement about data sharing; and the physician head of the other laboratory, who was also the project principal investigator (PI). In the end, he took us both to the university lawyers over this issue, who decided that the PI could do anything he wanted with the data.

This struggle involved a contradiction between two ways of viewing anthropological work. It also involved a trade-off between my own professional interest in publishing from data I had collected and the political utility of supporting the interests and assumptions of the PI. This no-win situation illustrates one of the dilemmas created by collapsing the worlds of "home" and "field" kept separate in the traditional narrative.

## What Do We Owe Our Informants?

Finally, I want to raise the question of what we owe our informants when we publish critiques of their practice. Of particular concern is the possibility that what we write may do them damage. After all, critique is presumably intended to change our informants' practice. One way or another it may have that effect, in the extreme case by putting them out of business. For some anthropological critics, that may indeed be the point of the exercise (a goal that itself requires ethical discussion.) For others, however, among whom I number myself, the point of critique is not to put our informants out of business but rather to suggest alternative ways to achieve their own goals. What concerns me is that critique so intended may be read differently by others and may be used for purposes we do not intend.

I showed my papers to my former laboratory head before submitting them for publication. In the year since my departure from his lab, I have continued this practice. So far, he has expressed no objection to my critiques of practice in his own and related laboratories and has requested only a few tiny changes of wording. While he comments that my papers make him feel "a bit uncomfortable," he insists that critique is good for the field and that they should be published. However, I worry that some others in the field may see this work as damaging. Both my informants and their competitors can read what I write. Could my work create a cost to the former of which they are unaware?

DISCUSSION

I have argued that in studying up in the United States, the juxtaposition of home and field, the movement of anthropologists to bases outside academic anthropology, the changing nature of funding, and the reversal in power relations all change the nature of fieldwork. I have suggested that these changes increase the mutual vulnerability of anthropologists and informants. They also create some new (or, in some cases, new versions of old) moral and practical dilemmas for fieldworkers.

This paper is work in progress: I am still thinking about what would be useful and appropriate to say about such dilemmas, and I welcome feedback. Obviously, this is a highly reflexive project. Not only do I attempt to turn the anthropological gaze upon the doing of anthropology itself, but my own fieldwork also involves people with whom I have much in common. My comments of course reflect the particularities of my own experience of studying up in science and technology.

I offer several points for discussion. First, although students continue to be taught the traditional narrative, it is obvious that a good deal of fieldwork these days no longer fits this story. We need some new narratives. Second, there has long been a tendency to treat anthropologists based outside the academy and colleagues whose field is not distant as not doing "real anthropology." This is unjust. What many of these innovative and entrepreneurial colleagues are doing is studying up, and, as Nader has shown, this is important work. It is high time for us to broaden our notions of what it means to have a "real" career in anthropology.

Studying up is not only important, it is also risky. As I have tried to show, to critique the practice of powerful people not only risks ethical and political quandaries, it may also involve risks to one's own professional future. My own work used to be funded by the medical informatics institute at the National Institutes of Health; after publishing critiques, which they have seen, I am unlikely to be funded by them again. Those who study up need recognition and understanding from their own discipline. After sticking one's neck out to critique the powerful, particularly from an untenured position, one needs such support.

Studying up is also risky to our informants. I am troubled by how cavalier some writers of ethnographic critique seem to be about the personal and professional vulnerability of the people they study. In fairness, I should note that this comment refers largely not to trained anthropologists but to people from other disciplines in science and technology studies who undertake ethnography without also taking on the associated philosophical and ethical stance (see Nyce and Lowgren 1995). I have heard papers about scientists and consumers of science that could only be called informant-bashing. In my view, doing fieldwork involves an ethical obligation to treat our informants with respect, whether or not we share their point of view. We who investigate elite people and agencies should remember that the possession of power alone does not justify willful damage.

At the same time, anthropology needs to come to terms with the phenomenon of powerful informants who read and contest our representations of them. A well-known anthropologist of science was attacked in both the popular and the social science press when she published an excellent book that analyzed her informants' work in terms they would not have chosen themselves. If we really believe that anthropologists can validly have a very different perspective than our informants, then we need to reaffirm that point when members of the communities studied are asked to review anthropological work about them. Furthermore, I suspect that those who study up experience a double standard. Anthropologists of science and technology are often subject to the judgments of their informants; for example, when I applied last year for an anthropology position at a university in California, several people from my latest lab were asked to write letters about me. In contrast, anthropologists who work in more traditional field sites are not normally subject to review by their informants. If such review is appropriate, then perhaps we should apply it more widely. If it is not, then I would urge caution in inviting elite, non-relativist informants to pass judgment on the publications, proposals, and unrelated job applications of anthropologists who study them.

A good deal has been written about the importance of accountability to our informants. Studying up—particularly from an untenured position—provides one with an opportunity to encounter the reality of doing ethnographic research in the absence of anthropological privilege. My own experience is that however much one might support this in theory—and I do—some kinds of "accountability" to one's informants can be difficult to live with. If we are going to treat the idea of cultural critique as normative, as it is these days in science and technology studies, we need to address some of these questions about the possible consequences of critiquing powerful people on their home ground.

# CHAPTER NINE

# Studying Those Who Study Us: Medical Informatics Appropriates Ethnography

In a previous paper (ch. 8) I distinguished between what I called the traditional and the new fieldwork narratives.[1] In the traditional fieldwork story, the anthropologist goes "away" to some distant site in a different social world and attempts to assimilate the knowledge and skills of relatively less powerful informants. What the latter make of the fieldworker's knowledge and skills has rarely been part of the story.

As anthropologists have turned to the study of technoscience, however, the balance of political and epistemological power on the fieldwork boundary has shifted. Anthropologists who study science and technology now work with (and often for) powerful informants who are well educated, competitive, and located in social worlds very close to home. Often knowledge workers themselves, they may be as interested in the anthropologist's research methods as she is in theirs. In this new fieldwork narrative, the researcher may be acutely aware that as she seeks to make sense of what she sees of her informants' work, this process is also taking place in the other direction.

In this paper, I describe one instance of this state of affairs and explore some of its consequences. I will draw upon my own extended participant observation in medical informatics, a field at the intersection of computer science and medicine. Focusing on border crossing (Traweek 1992) in an epistemological sense, I call attention to some unexpected trafficking across the boundary between informants and anthropologists "studying up" (Nader 1972, 1977, 1980) in technoscience: the appropriation by software designers of the ethnographic concepts and methods that anthropologists have been using to study them.

I will begin with some background material.

ETHNOGRAPHIC INVESTIGATIONS OF MEDICAL INFORMATICS

Computers have been applied to problems in medicine for several decades. For the past two decades, anthropologists and other social scientists have applied ethnographic techniques to supporting—and sometimes investigating—this endeavor. The first full-length anthropological study of system implementation in medical informatics was Lundsgaarde's pioneering evaluation of the PROMIS system (Fischer, Stratmann, Lundsgaarde, and Steele 1987; Lundsgaarde, Fischer, and Steele 1981). Fieldwork took place from 1976–77; the book was published in 1981. There is now a considerable literature derived from ethnographic studies, addressing such themes as the nature of knowledge in different medical fields (Nyce and Graves 1990), workplace organization and practice (Fafchamps 1991; Fafchamps, Young, and Tang 1991; Kaplan and Duchon 1988), patient education (Forsythe 1995), ethnographic contributions to system design (Nyce and Timpka 1993), and evaluation of medical information systems (Forsythe and Buchanan 1991; Kaplan and Maxwell 1994; Lundsgaarde 1987). Much of this work has been published in journals and proceedings read by people in medical computing.

Informaticians have two apparently contradictory responses to these contributions to their field by social scientists. First, they routinely delete them. Although anthropology is considerably older than medical informatics and anthropologists have been working in informatics for quite a while, informaticians habitually refer to ethnography as "new," "soft," and "unscientific." The products of ethnographic work in medical informatics tend to be overlooked. At a December 1995 meeting on evaluation at an agency of the National Institutes of Health (NIH), for example, a forthcoming book by two "old boys" in the field was repeatedly referred to as "the first book on evaluation in medical informatics," despite the prior existence of two books on the same topic by social scientists (Anderson, Aydin, and Jay 1994; Lundsgaarde, Fischer, and Steele 1981).[2] One of these books was actually being advertised at the meeting.

In apparent contrast to this tendency to delete social scientific contributions to medical informatics, professionals in medical computing have recently begun to attempt such studies themselves. In the early 1990s, apparently inspired by publications by social scientists,[3] informaticians began to undertake and publish surveys (Gorman, Ash, and Wykoff 1994; Gorman and Helfand 1995). More recently, informaticians have taken up ethnography. The 1995 and 1996 proceedings of the American Medical Informatics Association (AMIA) meetings contain roughly half a dozen papers based on "ethnographic" and "observational" work by informaticians who are not social scientists (e.g., Coble, Maffitt, Orland, and Kahn 1995; Coiera 1996; Rosenal, Forsythe, Musen, and Seiver 1995; Tang, Jaworski, Fellencer, Kreider, LaRosa, and Marquardt 1996; Tang, Jaworski, Fellencer, LaRosa, Lassa, Lipsey, and Marquardt 1995).

These studies demonstrate their authors' conception of what surveys and ethnography entail. The result is sometimes disconcerting, especially in the case of the would-be ethnography; the latter tends to differ considerably from ethnography as anthropologists understand it. Equally disconcerting for anthropologists working in informatics has been the rapid change in funding patterns that has accompanied the development of this home-grown social science. The main NIH institute that supports medical informatics has funded several anthropologists over the years to carry out the "social" (often the evaluation) piece of system-building projects. As far as I know, this support has now ceased. Instead, the institute is funding physicians and computer scientists with no social science training to carry out new, "more scientific" versions of social science research, invented by informaticians looking back across the border at ethnographers studying them.

This situation is ironic, since it is in part the outcome of years of effort by social scientists to get informaticians to see our applied ethnographic skills as useful to them. Having introduced their informants to ethnography in the first place, anthropologists now find their potential contributions replaced by improvised versions of their own methods. This situation is also economically and professionally problematic to social scientists who have been dependent upon this funding and have developed specialized expertise in informatics-related research.

INFORMATICIANS CONSTRUCT ETHNOGRAPHY

Professionals in medical informatics include physicians, nurses, medical librarians, computer scientists, and information scientists. Of these, the most influential in shaping the field are physicians, some of whom also have doctorates in computer science. Least influential are nurses and medical librarians (see ch. 11), a fact of relevance here because these are also likely to be the individuals with the most exposure to qualitative research.

Many informaticians have had some acquaintance with ethnography from reading publications that draw on ethnographic research, hearing talks at professional meetings, working with social scientists on research teams, and/ or being subjects of ethnographic inquiry themselves. They naturally bring to the understanding of this research method theories of knowledge, assumptions, and practices derived from their own professional training. Elsewhere, I have attempted to characterize something of the intellectual worldview of informaticians (chs. 1–3; Forsythe and Buchanan 1991). Here I will mention only a few things. They tend to be positivists, committed to what they think of as "hard science." They tend to share the medical model of research as requiring randomized, controlled clinical trials that involve double-blinding and thus often exclude consideration of subjective experience. Informaticians equate "research" with "experiment" and "analysis" with "quantification." For many, the notion of "uncontrolled" research is an oxymoron; accounts of subjective experience, including publications by professional anthropologists, are dismissed as "anecdotal." Finally, many people in this field, particularly the physicians, have had no research training at all. Informaticians with doctorates in computing sciences have been trained in research but in a tradition in which "research" means building a software prototype. To sum up, these are people with a strong bias in favor of a positivist image of science, but very little real-world research experience that might serve to temper that image. Few have had any training in social science.

How do informaticians understand ethnography? Below I offer some generalizations based on views I have heard articulated in the course of my fieldwork.

### *"Anyone Can Do Ethnography—It's Just a Matter of Common Sense!"*

Informaticians see ethnography as something that either requires no particular expertise or for which their present expertise already equips them. I cannot tell you the number of people in medical computing who, having read and found useful the product of social science research in their field (often one of our papers on physicians' information needs—Forsythe, Buchanan, Osheroff, and Miller 1992; Osheroff, Forsythe, Buchanan, Bankowitz, Blumenfeld, and Miller 1991), then asked me to suggest "just one article" to enable them to do ethnography themselves.

During the early years of my fieldwork, I responded with earnest explanations intended to convey that they hadn't quite understood. I would point out gently that ethnography involved understanding a good deal of theory in order to achieve a particular conceptual stance in relation to the subject. For this reason, reading just one article wouldn't do the trick; they would have to read at least a whole book, and hopefully a good deal more.

The response was invariably some version of "forget the theory, just tell me the techniques." The notion that anthropology's strongest technique is its philosophical stance makes little sense to positivists. Sticking with that argument sounds hostile to them and can produce a hostile response. Stressing the need for formal training sounds like refusal to help, that is, refusal to divulge those simple techniques that would enable them to do ethnography on their own. My final suggestion that they work with a trained anthropologist was often understood as self-seeking, an attempt to try to protect the jobs of social scientists like me. I can count on the fingers of one hand the informaticians who actually heard and took seriously the argument as I meant it. (One or two of them have now hired their own anthropologists.) Most have either begun to carry out do-it-yourself ethnography or have hired non-anthropologists (e.g., nurses, teachers, or epidemiologists) to take on the role of "house ethnographer" in their work groups.

Frustrated by the failure of my early attempts to explain how anthropologists see ethnography, I have recently begun to offer a blunter response—some version of "what would *you* say if I asked for the name of a single article on medicine so that I could take out your appendix?" Social scientists love this response, but physicians and computer scientists either react with fury or don't hear the point at all. What interests me about this state of affairs is the apparent invisibility of ethnographic expertise—very few computer scientists and physicians appear to believe that social scientific research takes any special knowledge at all. In contrast, informaticians take their *own* expertise very seriously. This tendency to emphasize their own expertise while overlooking that of social scientists is puzzling because of the overlap in the work of informaticians and anthropologists. Presumably this is the reason why many of them are interested in the first place in doing their own ethnography.

The view of ethnography as "simply a matter of common sense" implies that for informaticians, at least, it requires no special training to do it. In informatics, an M.D. after one's name is seen as qualifying one to do almost anything. Computer scientists share a similar confidence in their own intelligence. Informaticians routinely undertake with confidence research tasks that impinge on neighboring disciplines (e.g., linguistics), asserting (in the words of one informant), "We're smart people; we can do that." Ethnography strikes them as equally accessible.

From an anthropological standpoint, of course, ethnography is not just a matter of common sense. Indeed, it runs counter to common sense, since it requires one to identify and problematize things that insiders take for granted (and thus tend to overlook). It takes considerable time to produce a good fieldworker. In fact, it takes as long to train a good ethnographer as it does to produce an expert in medical diagnosis (an average of seven years for a Ph.D. in anthropology—presumably similar for qualitative sociology or history—plus several years of real-world experience).

## *"Being Insiders Qualifies Medical Professionals to Do Ethnography in Medical Settings"*

Informaticians assume their insider status to be an advantage, since they believe they know what is going on in medical settings. From an anthropological standpoint, insiders do not make the best observers of a social situation. In fact, we tend to believe that ethnography works best when conducted by an outsider with considerable inside experience. The reason is that we see the ethnographer's job as not to replicate the insiders' perspective but rather to elicit and *analyze* it in the light of systematic comparison between inside and outside views of the situation. This includes detecting tacit knowledge, something that by definition is generally invisible to insiders. As anthropologists understand it, the ethnographic stance requires mental distance. Medical providers may indeed be very familiar with their practice settings, but such inside knowledge is not the same thing as a systematic overview of a situation.

## *"Since Ethnography Does Not Involve Randomized Clinical Trials, It Involves No Systematic Method at All"*

Informaticians equate scientific research with randomized trials, double-blinding, and quantitative analysis. They take the anthropological reliance on qualitative analysis and subjective experience, and our tendency to avoid "controlled experiments" and preformulated "research instruments," to imply the absence of any research method. In other words, they place ethnography in the realm of the "anecdotal," the term with which they normally dismiss evidence viewed as unscientific. The interpretation of the more improvisational ethnographic approach as a complete absence of method may also reflect the intentional unobtrusiveness of ethnographic inquiry, which may be invisible to an untrained eye. (With respect to the latter point, anthropologists' success in fitting into medical settings without drawing attention to themselves with disruptive data-gathering methods may work against informaticians' recognition of them as scientific colleagues.) In any case, since informaticians see ethnography as the antithesis of scientific method, their approach to doing it sometimes amounts to "anything goes."

## "Doing Fieldwork Is Just Talking to People and Reporting What They Say"

Viewing qualitative research as anecdotal in nature, informaticians understand ethnography as "just talking to people and reporting what they say" —perhaps equivalent to journalism. Presumably this is what they experience when fieldworkers study them or do ethnography on their behalf; the selectivity of question-asking and observation, and the process of inferential data analysis are invisible to them as informants and research colleagues. Fieldwork does of course involve talking to people, but to anthropologists this is no more the entire task than system-building is "just typing" or medical diagnosis is "just talking to patients." The important point is what one is *doing* when typing or talking. Competent fieldworkers do not take what people say at face value; they treat people's views as *data*, not results, just as what patients say about their condition is not the same thing as medical diagnosis. The job of the social scientist includes understanding and analyzing what people say, but this is not always apparent to informaticians.

## "To Find Out What People Do, Just Ask Them!"

Many people in medical informatics and cognitive science treat verbal representations as congruent with and predictive of what takes place "on the ground" (chs. 2, 3). They also tend to assume that human patterns of action in the world are consistent over time. This accounts for the widespread reliance on "think aloud" narratives (which are taken as accurate descriptions of human problem-solving) and for the tendency to move from a very small number of cases to general statements about how the human mind works. When informaticians undertake ethnography, they act on the basis of these assumptions; this leads them to take for granted that what people say is what they will do, and that if people do something once or twice they will always do it. As the AMIA papers reveal, informaticians treat focus groups and short-term (e.g., two hour) synchronic observation as revealing general patterns of human action.

For anthropologists, in contrast, the predictive value of verbal representations and the generality of short-term observation are seen as questionable. Ethnography does of course entail eliciting people's understandings of their own and others' behavior, but only the most naive of fieldworkers treats such understandings as necessarily constituting reliable data about systematic patterns of action. Anthropologists see the relation between representation and visible action as complex (Geertz 1973, 1983) and know from our observational tradition that people's verbal representations of their own behavior are often partial and sometimes incorrect.

## *"Observational Research Is Just a Matter of Looking and Listening to Find the Patterns Out There"*

Informaticians seem to believe that social and organizational patterns are visible and audible; one need only look and listen to detect them. This first became clear to me when I overheard a physician characterize my role in observing hospital work rounds as being "a walking tape recorder." As it happened, I had tried carrying a tape recorder for several days for that project and taped the work rounds. The resultant audiotapes contained an indecipherable babble from which this physician's highly competent secretary was unable to create a meaningful transcript. In contrast, on the basis of my written fieldnotes, I consistently produced readable transcripts with additional analytical comments. The physician's construction of this situation was to see me as a better sort of tape recorder, ostensibly because I had legs. (Actually, the original tape recorder, in effect, had legs as well, since I had carried it around.) My role in selecting and interpreting the information that I recorded, and in compiling the data into narrative accounts, was completely invisible to the physician, perhaps because he experienced morning work rounds as unproblematically ordered.

This positivist vision of ethnography leads informaticians to believe that an audio- or a videorecording itself constitutes qualitative analysis. For example, the informatics review board at the NIH once urged me to include videotaping in a proposal for a year-long ethnographic study of emergency medicine.

Overlooking the ethical and legal issues that the suggestion was bound to raise for hospital authorities, not to mention the question of how and when I would analyze a year's worth of videotapes, they clearly felt that the addition of video technology would make my fieldwork more scientific and reliable.

From an anthropological standpoint, of course, this view reflects a misunderstanding. Patterns of human thought and action are no more visible than the diagnosis of an individual's illness. To imagine that behavioral patterns become visible and self-explanatory in a videotape is analogous to suggesting that a photograph reveals the diagnosis of a patient's illness. It may be that a skilled physician can diagnose certain maladies from a photograph, just as a skilled social scientist picks up patterns from analyzing audio- and videorecordings. But in both cases, the expertise is in the mind and technique of the analyst, not in the recording of the events. What this positivist perspective overlooks is the selectivity and interpretation that go into the processes of data-gathering and analysis.

The way informaticians make sense of ethnography will not surprise anthropologists of science, technology, and medicine. Anyone who has carried out fieldwork in technoscientific worlds is surely familiar with the contrasting visions of data-gathering and interpretation that grow out of positivist and relativist perspectives as well as the difficulty positivism has in seeing relativism in its own terms. Informaticians' construction of ethnography is clearly based on some assumptions not shared by most anthropologists.

INSTANTIATING THE POSITIVIST VISION OF ETHNOGRAPHY

What do informaticians actually do when they set out to do ethnography? As I mentioned above, recent proceedings of the annual AMIA conference contain papers in which non–social scientists have applied their own interpretations of ethnography, variously referred to as "ethnography," "ethnographically derived methods," or "observational methods" (Coble, Maffit, Orland, and Kahn 1995; Coiera 1996; Rosenal, Forsythe, Musen, and Seiver 1995; Tang, Jaworski, Fellencer, Kreider, LaRosa, and Marquardt 1996; Tang, Jaworski, Fellencer, LaRosa, Lassa, Lipsey, and Marquardt 1995). Several of these authors are people I have known as informants for many years. I base the following discussion on having heard each of these papers presented, on discussions with some of the authors, and (in the case of the Rosenal paper) on my own knowledge of the project.

First, it is instructive to note what the authors of these papers report having done. Rosenal and colleagues carried out 44 hours of observations in a critical care unit of a university hospital over a period of one month. In addition, they interviewed five people.[4] In their 1995 study, Tang and colleagues report having shadowed 30 clinicians for two to four hours each, for a total of 78 hours. The team also interviewed 30 clinicians. In the 1996 study, Tang and colleagues observed a total of 38 clinicians over seven sites for two hours each. They also interviewed 33 people. Coiera reports having undertaken 23 "preliminary semi-structured interviews" and shadowing twelve people for four hours each. Finally, Coble and colleagues (1995) report having carried out approximately 300 hours of interviewing and videotaping for a study of "physicians' true needs," using a method called "contextual inquiry."

Except in the case of Coble's study (in which it is unclear how much of that 300 hours was devoted to interviewing as opposed to videotaping), these are rather small numbers. Shadowing people for a total of two to four hours each is very short-term observation, especially for a fieldworker with little or no previous observational experience.

None of these authors appears to have had any serious ethnographic or anthropological training. Rosenal is a physician specializing in critical care medicine. He was inspired to try to do ethnography himself by having read some of my own papers. His ethnographic training was limited to several discussions with me during a term spent at my university. Tang is a physician who in a past job led a design team that contained a trained ethnographer, Fafchamps. In his present position, he has assembled a group of nurses whom he directs in carrying out a new, more "scientific" form of ethnography that owes something to industrial engineering. Coiera has a Ph.D. in computer science. Finally, Coble has had (as far as I know) no training in either social science or medicine. The head of her research team is a physician whom I knew as an informant during his graduate training in informatics. At the 1995 AMIA meeting, he told me proudly, "Now we have someone like you" (meaning Coble). When I inquired about her training in social science, he looked mystified; later, Coble told me that she had learned the method of "contextual inquiry" from a weekend workshop conducted by a social scientist.

The "ethnographic" research carried out by these individuals has considerable credibility within the medical informatics community. It was presented at the main professional meeting of this community and appears in the peer-reviewed proceedings. The work of one of these teams (Tang) is supported by NIH. On the basis of what qualifications is this home-grown social science taken so seriously? From the above examples, it appears that for a physician or computer scientist, sufficient qualification is conferred by having talked with, worked with, or simply read the writing of a trained ethnographer. The rest is apparently a matter of "common sense."

While several of these neo-ethnographers refer knowledgeably to the richness of their "ethnographic" findings (Tang in particular has mastered the vocabulary of social science), from an anthropological standpoint they do very little with the relatively small amount of observational and inter-view data they collected. (Coble et al. apparently collected a good deal of data.) A major strength of ethnography is its ability to uncover tacit assumptions, thus making them available for questioning and testing. As Nyce and Lowgren (1995) have noted, however, informaticians tend to borrow ethnographic data-gathering techniques without also borrowing (or understanding) the conceptual structure from which they derive. Since decontextualizing ethnographic techniques in this way reduces their analytical power, the resultant "insider ethnography" takes local meanings at face value, overlooking tacit assumptions rather than questioning them. None of these "ethnographic" studies by informaticians raises problems of epistemology or meaning, although anthropologists working in informatics invariably encounter and report such issues when doing ethnography in similar settings. Instead, the informatician ethnographers seem simply to quantify everything they can, supporting their findings with copious statistics and pie charts.

From my standpoint, these analyses are superficial. They certainly lack the critical perspective that many anthropologists working in technoscience derive from their ethnographic work. However, since the powerful "old boys" of medical informatics have not always welcomed critique of their assumptions, the absence of a critical edge in this "insider" ethnography probably makes it much more palatable from their standpoint. While this work may add little in terms of new understanding, it also does not rock the boat—something to which the old boys are rather sensitive.

DISCUSSION

I have described some epistemological and methodological trafficking across the fieldwork boundary between anthropology and medical informatics.

Over the past decade or two, social scientists have been busy on the anthropological side of the fence, constructing theories about our informants' practice. For at least some of this time, those informants have also been at work on their side of the boundary, building theories about what we do. Some social scientists have become players in the world of informatics, offering suggestions on how to improve the practice of system design; sometimes these suggestions contravene conventional truths of medical computing. On the other side of the border, some informaticians have begun to construct themselves as ethnographers, reconfiguring ethnography in ways that sometimes run counter to anthropological truths about what constitutes valid and meaningful research.

A struggle is taking place on the boundary between anthropology and medical informatics. At issue are the meaning of ethnography and what constitutes ethnographic expertise as well as what should be the source of authority in this domain. Who gets to define what counts as ethnography? Whose perspective should determine what counts as ethnographic expertise and as credible ethnographic research? This struggle extends to resources, as informaticians compete with social scientists for access to NIH funds to support social science research.

On a broader level, social scientists and informaticians are contesting the location of the disciplinary boundary that divides them. Anthropologists working in medical informatics still tend to identify themselves as anthropologists, but claim expertise in territory that informaticians see as their own. Conversely, informaticians conducting their versions of ethnographic research show no desire to be seen as anthropologists but rather seek to push the boundary of their own field into the realm of social science.

How should we react to this situation? My own reaction is complex; the case looks different depending on the position from which one views it. Intellectually, I am intrigued by the informant appropriation of ethnography. From a relativist perspective, I admire their creativity and enterprise. But I cannot view this case solely from a distance, since I happen to be implicated in the story. Some of the informaticians described in this paper learned about ethnography from me; my explanations, attempted demonstrations, and publications helped to create the conditions in which they decided to try it themselves. And then there is the question of money. I was paid to do ethnographic studies in medical informatics; as this appropriation has become a trend, my own research funds have dried up. Committed as I am intellectually to a relativist perspective, the appropriation of ethnography in medical informatics threatens my own interests and those of other soft-money anthropologists in a similar position.

This brings me back to the theme with which this paper began: the huge difference for the researcher between the old and the new fieldwork narratives as contexts for field research. The phenomenon of appropriation by informants sounds very different against the background of these two narratives.

The traditional fieldwork story grants epistemological privilege to the anthropologist. Writing about distant people less powerful than she, the traditional fieldworker holds all the representational cards. Her understanding of her informants' work practice generally becomes—in our literature, at least—the uncontested account of what is really going on.

Consider a reversal of this state of affairs taking place in the context of the traditional fieldwork story. Imagine a group of marginalized, indigenous peoples in the Third World who begin to appropriate and reconfigure ethnographic methods picked up from their anthropologist, applying them autonomously in their own milieu in pursuit of social justice. Surely any anthropologist would be delighted to have been the source (however unwittingly) of tactics that such informants could apply to improve their own situation. Disparities between the informants' construal of ethnography and more usual anthropological understandings of it could be waved away (or even celebrated) under the flag of cultural relativism.

Contrast that with the case presented in this paper: the same basic plot, but this time set in the context of the new fieldwork narrative. Instead of powerless informants located in some conveniently distant corner of the world, we have powerful physicians and computer scientists, willing and able to resist if they don't like what the anthropologist writes about them (see ch. 8). Instead of independently funded researchers heading back from time-bounded field sessions toward the security of home and tenure, we have soft-money anthropologists trying to survive for long periods of time in their informants' world by making themselves useful to bosses and colleagues in technoscience. In the context of this new fieldwork narrative, in which epistemological and other power relations are reversed, the tale of ethnographic appropriation becomes a different story. Whereas under traditional conditions the informants' use of ethnography poses no threat to the anthropologist, the same act by informants in technoscience sets up competition between them and the anthropologist.

Obviously, more is at stake for the anthropologist in this second version. Informaticians' appropriation of the ethnographic method and their move to redefine (within the realm of medical informatics, at least) what counts as ethnographic expertise bring them into direct competition with their anthropologists for federal funding for *social science* research. This is a struggle that the anthropologists are unlikely to win. Conceptual and methodological weaknesses that a social scientist might find in the informaticians' "ethnographic" proposals are not apparent to the clinicians and computer professionals on the review board.

Informants' agreement with our interpretations of their lives and actions has never been required of anthropologists working under traditional fieldwork conditions. Under those conditions, it has never really mattered much what they made of our work. Thus, we could freely affirm our informants' right to construct us and our research techniques as they wished. In the study of technoscience, however, exercise of this right is having significant consequences for the fieldworkers. Anthropologists doing ethnographic work in medical informatics have provided their informants with a new vocabulary and set of methods that the scientists have been able to reconfigure, adapt to their own paradigmatic base, and turn to their own ends.

Ironically, anthropologists working in medical informatics find themselves hoist with their own petard. Having spent a decade or two trying to persuade informaticians that their ethnographic skills enable them to make a valuable contribution to the design and evaluation of medical information systems, anthropologists now find themselves replaced in job slots and research budgets by physicians, computer scientists, and a variety of other non–social scientists practicing home-grown social science. The attempt to demonstrate that ethnographic approaches can usefully be applied in informatics has clearly been successful. However, that success has simply created a new arena in which more powerful informaticians are out-competing anthropologists for resources. Social scientists appear to have won the battle but lost the war.

# CHAPTER TEN

# "It's Just a Matter of Common Sense": Ethnography as Invisible Work

Many people look to computerized technologies to help solve problems of information access and management in work settings.[1] If computer systems are to achieve this goal, their developers need detailed knowledge about both information-related problems and the nature of the settings in which these problems occur. Questions about work-related problems and their organizational contexts extend into the realm of the social. As the design world increasingly recognizes, social scientists can contribute to the development of more usable technical tools by providing useful answers to these questions. One research approach that has demonstrated utility in this context is ethnography, used for over a century by anthropologists and qualitative sociologists to illuminate real-world work processes and work settings.

Ethnography is useful at all stages of system development and evaluation. Since Lundsgaarde's pioneering work in the 1970s (Lundsgaarde, Fischer, and Steele 1981), the application of ethnographic research skills to aspects of software design and evaluation developed gradually through the 1980s. There is now a substantial literature on the subject (Blomberg, Giacomi, Mosher, and Swenton-Wall 1993; Fafchamps 1991; Forsythe 1995; Forsythe and Buchanan 1991; Lundsgaarde 1987; Nyce and Timpka 1993; Suchman 1987, 1995; Nardi 1997).

Early applications of ethnographic skills in software design and evaluation were generally viewed as experimental, at least on the part of computer scientists and engineers. Over time, however, many members of the development community have come to see the utility of ethnographic input to design. The computer-supported cooperative work (CSCW) community has been particularly open to the addition of anthropological perspectives and methods to the development tool kit (Galegher and Kraut 1990). By the mid-1990s, ethnography was becoming established as a useful skill in technology design.

As this message has become accepted, corporations and research laboratories have employed anthropologists to take part in the development process. In addition, growing numbers of non-anthropologists have begun attempting to borrow ethnographic techniques. The results of this borrowing have brought out into the open a kind of paradox: ethnography looks and sounds straightforward—easily borrowed, in fact. However, this is not really the case. The work of untrained ethnographers tends to overlook things that anthropologists see as important parts of the research process (Nyce and Lowgren 1995). The consistency of this pattern suggests that some aspects of ethnographic fieldwork are invisible to the untrained eye. In short, ethnography would appear to present us with an example of invisible work.

In the sections below, I explore this phenomenon, drawing on my own decade of experience as an anthropologist using ethnographic methods to investigate and support design in artificial intelligence and medical informatics. Comparing the way ethnographic research is understood by anthropologists with examples of the application of quasi-ethnographic techniques by people from other disciplines, I attempt to unravel which aspects of ethnographic expertise are invisible and to explore why they seem to be overlooked.

WHAT IS ETHNOGRAPHY?

Ethnography as a research process entails the use of three elements in combination. First, fieldworkers make use of a set of ethnographic data-gathering methods that include participant observation, formal and informal interviewing, and sometimes also analysis of documentary sources (Powdermaker 1966; Wax 1971; Werner and Schoepfle 1987). Flexible and unobtrusive, these field methods were designed for use in uncontrolled (and uncontrollable) real-life settings. In use, they enable the fieldworker to detect consistent patterns of thought and practice and to investigate the relationship between them—an important comparison, since what people do is not always the same as what they say they do.

Second, these methods are grounded in theory, as are the methods anthropologists use to analyze their field data. The large body of literature in anthropology and qualitative sociology provides a theoretical framework for distinguishing between different sorts of knowledge and for investigating the relationship between beliefs and action in social situations. The cross-cultural ethnographic record also provides a kind of testbed against which to compare particular findings and to evaluate general theories about human traits.

And third, anthropologists apply these methods in the context of a distinctive philosophical stance. Based in social science theory and intended to help researchers to take as little as possible for granted, this ethnographic stance promotes the conceptual distance necessary for systematic comparison of multiple perspectives on events and processes.

Ethnography produces in-depth understanding of real-world social processes. Properly done, it provides detailed insight into the concepts and premises that underlie what people do—but that they are often unaware of. The power of ethnography as a research approach derives from use of the data-gathering methods together with the philosophical stance and the conceptual structure in which they are grounded. In general, ethnographic fieldworkers do not use preformulated research instruments. Instead, the fieldworker herself is the research instrument, one which is "calibrated" first through training in theory and methodology and then through experience.

Learning to *do* ethnography involves learning to *see* social situations in a way that problematizes certain phenomena. It also involves learning to maintain careful epistemological discipline. Such attention to disciplining the researcher may sound easy compared to research methods that focus instead on controlling the research subjects and/or the context in which they appear. However, field research is by no means straightforward: it takes talent, training, and practice to become a competent field researcher and careful data collection and analysis to produce reliable results. As with any kind of skill, what makes ethnography look easy is expertise.

## CLARIFYING THE NATURE OF ETHNOGRAPHIC EXPERTISE

The philosophical tradition from which ethnography derives is somewhat different from the philosophical tradition that underlies the natural sciences, computer science, cognitive psychology, and engineering. The former is known to social scientists as relativism, the latter as realism or positivism. In part because of this difference in underlying philosophy, practitioners from science and medicine often misconstrue what anthropological fieldworkers are doing. Such differences in perspective can be difficult for positivists to see and discuss, however, because many scientists do not realize that they have been trained in a distinct philosophical tradition. Below, I illustrate the implications of these differences in perspective by addressing six common misconceptions that I have encountered in working on software design projects.

## Six Misconceptions about the Use of Ethnography in Design

1. Anyone can do ethnography—it's just a matter of common sense.
2. Being insiders qualifies people to do ethnography in their own work setting.
3. Since ethnography does not involve preformulated study designs, it involves no systematic method at all—"anything goes."
4. Doing fieldwork is just chatting with people and reporting what they say.
5. To find out what people do, just ask them!
6. Behavioral and organizational patterns exist "out there" in the world; observational research is just a matter of looking and listening to detect these patterns.

## Correction

1. Anyone can do ethnography: Many technical people see ethnography as something that either requires no particular expertise or for which their present expertise already equips them. To them, it's "just a matter of common sense." Actually, ethnography runs counter to common sense, since it requires one to identify and problematize things that insiders take for granted (and thus tend to overlook). It takes a good deal of training and experience to learn to do this. It may also take courage on occasion, since insiders tend to experience their own assumptions as obvious truths. The lone anthropologist in a technical or other field site may be the only one to question these truths.

2. Being insiders qualifies people to do ethnography in their own work setting: The assumption that senior insiders make the best observers of a social situation informs the "expert" model used in knowledge acquisition for software development (ch. 2; Buchanan, Barstow, Bechtal, Bennett, Clancey, Kulikowski, Mitchell, and Waterman 1983; Forsythe and Buchanan 1989). However, competence as an insider does not make one an accurate observer. In fact, ethnography usually works best when conducted by an *outsider with considerable inside experience*. The reason is that the ethnographer's job is not to replicate the insiders' perspective but rather to elicit and *analyze* it through systematic comparison between inside and outside views of

particular events and processes. This task includes detecting tacit knowledge, something that by definition is generally invisible to insiders. The ethnographic stance requires mental distance. Insiders do indeed know what is going on in their practice settings, but such inside knowledge is not the same thing as a systematic and analytical overview of the situation (see example below).

3. Since ethnography does not involve preformulated study designs, it involves no systematic method at all: People trained in the natural sciences tend to equate scientific research with randomized controlled trials, double-blinding, and quantitative analysis. They take the anthropological reliance on qualitative analysis and subjective experience, as well as the tendency to avoid "controlled experiments" and rigid, preset "research instruments," to imply the absence of any research method. In other words, they place ethnography in the realm of the "anecdotal," the term with which they normally dismiss evidence viewed as unscientific. The interpretation of the more improvisational ethnographic approach as a complete absence of method may also reflect the intentional unobtrusiveness of ethnographic inquiry, which may be invisible to an untrained eye. (With respect to the latter point, anthropologists' success in fitting into work settings without drawing attention to themselves with disruptive data-gathering methods may work against the recognition of them in technical circles as scientific colleagues.) In any case, since non-anthropologists often perceive ethnography as devoid of scientific method, their own approach to trying it sometimes amounts to "anything goes."

In contrast, anthropologists see ethnographic work as technical in nature and take seriously issues of methodological appropriateness, procedure, and validity (Werner and Schoepfle 1987). Proper ethnography involves systematic method and epistemological discipline, neither of which is seen by anthropologists as necessarily requiring rigid adherence to preformulated research protocols. Qualitative researchers are wary of preformulated questionnaires because they often turn out to ask the wrong questions, just as so-called "controlled experiments" don't always tell us much about complex social behavior. In doing ethnography, initial research questions are carefully refined and pursued as fieldwork develops. When field anthropologists discover that they have been asking the wrong questions, they adjust their research formulation in the course of a study. Experienced anthropologists learn to expect such mid-course corrections (Rosaldo 1993: 7) and value the increased accuracy they produce. While it certainly differs from so-called "controlled" research, ethnography is nevertheless a matter of careful, conscious method.

4. Doing fieldwork is just chatting with people: Viewing qualitative research as anecdotal in nature, people trained in the sciences often understand ethnography as "just talking to people and reporting what they say" —perhaps equivalent to transcription. Presumably this is what they experience when fieldworkers study them or do ethnography on their behalf; the selectivity of question-asking and observation and the process of inferential data analysis are invisible to them as informants and research colleagues. Doing fieldwork certainly involves talking to people, but this is no more the entire task than system-building is "just typing" or medical diagnosis is "just talking to patients." The important point is what one is *doing* when typing or talking. Competent fieldworkers do not take what people say at face value; they treat people's views as *data*, not results, just as what patients say about their condition is not the same thing as medical diagnosis. The job of the social scientist is to *understand and analyze* what people say. Perhaps because the uninitiated see only the fieldworker's interaction with her respondents and do not see the analytical expertise being deployed at the same time, they may assume that they already have the skills to carry out ethnographic fieldwork.

5. To know what people do, just ask them: Many people in the cognitive sciences treat verbal representations as congruent with and predictive of what takes place "on the ground" (chs. 2, 3). They also tend to assume that human patterns of action in the world are consistent over time. This accounts for the widespread reliance on "think aloud" and "cognitive walk through" narratives (which are taken as accurate descriptions of human problem-solving) and for the tendency to move from a very small number of cases to general statements about how the human mind works. When non-anthropologists undertake ethnography, they act on the basis of these assumptions; this leads them to take for granted that what people say is what they will do, and that if people do something once or twice they will always do it. The resultant approach treats focus groups and short-term (e.g., two hour) synchronic observation as revealing general patterns of human action.

For anthropologists, in contrast, the predictive value of verbal representations and the generality of short-term observation are questionable. Ethnography does of course entail eliciting people's understandings of their own and others' behavior, but only the most naive of fieldworkers would treat such understandings as reliable data about systematic behavioral patterns. Anthropologists see the relation between representation and visible action as complex (Geertz 1973, 1983) and know from our observational tradition that people's verbal representations of their own behavior are often partial and sometimes incorrect. In other words, it is imperative to watch people engaged in activity as well as to ask them about it. Such observations in classical ethnography tend to be quite extended—a matter of months or years. While observational periods may be much shorter in the design context, they are still extremely useful when conducted by a competent observer. In system evaluation, for example, it is advisable to observe people using the system as well as to elicit their opinions about it. Focus groups and surveys are no substitute for the combination of participant observation and interview data.

6. Behavioral and organizational patterns exist "out there" in the world: Observational research is sometimes perceived by others as just a matter of looking to see what is "out there." Many technical people seem to assume that social and organizational patterns are visible and audible; one need only look and listen to detect them. This leads them to imagine that an audio- or videorecording itself constitutes qualitative analysis. This is a misunderstanding. Patterns of human thought and action are no more visible than the diagnosis of an individual's illness. To imagine that behavioral patterns become visible and self-explanatory in a videotape is analogous to believing that a photograph reveals the diagnosis of a patient's illness. It may be that a skilled physician can diagnose certain maladies from a photograph, just as a skilled social scientist picks up patterns from analyzing audio- and videorecordings. But in both cases, the expertise is in the mind and technique of the analyst, not in the recording itself. What this common misconception fails to grasp is the selectivity and interpretation that go into the process of gathering careful ethnographic data, writing useful fieldnotes (Emerson, Fretz, and Shaw 1995; Sanjek 1990), and analyzing the data in an appropriate and systematic way.

APPLYING THESE MISCONCEPTIONS

I have described some misconceptions about ethnographic methods that I have encountered among software designers (and others). As these points suggest, people untrained in anthropology or qualitative sociology may overlook important aspects of ethnographic work. These include the understanding that doing ethnography requires expertise; that analyzing a social situation entails much more than just having "inside" familiarity with that situation; that ethnographic research involves the application of conscious method that—while unobtrusive—is systematic and theory-based; that people's self-reports about their own and each other's actions are not taken at face value by anthropologists, but rather are systematically tested against other self-reports and against observable behavior; that seasoned fieldworkers carry out a good deal of observation and amass considerable data before producing generalizations about social patterns; and that good social analysis is the product of careful selection and thoughtful interpretation. When people from other disciplines attempt to borrow ethnographic research techniques, the result often fails to manifest these principles.

## Examples

To illustrate the types of difficulties caused by relying on the misconceptions described above, I will offer two examples in the sections below. First, perhaps the most widespread strategy adopted by would-be ethnographers is Misconception no. 5: "If you want to know what people do, just ask them." This commonsense approach to social research is liable to produce unreliable data when used on its own. The problem is that human beings—no matter how expert—rarely possess a broad overview of the social practices in which they engage. Since they tend not to be aware of this, however, they may believe that they are providing accurate data when they are not. To illustrate this, I will contrast an expert's reconstruction of a familiar social process with observational data on the same process.

Second, to illustrate the characteristic superficiality of "do-it-yourself" ethnography, I will describe some recent quasi-ethnographic work in medical informatics. This work overlooks the epistemological and methodological challenges that ethnographic methods are intended to address. These include:

1. The problem of perspective—understanding what events mean to the actors themselves, as opposed to what they might mean if the fieldworker had done them. The epistemological discipline that constitutes an essential part of the ethnographic method requires maintaining a scrupulous and systematic distinction between the knowledge and assumptions) of particular informants (or categories of informants) and the knowledge and assumptions of the observer(s). To fail to pay attention to this issue is

to take for granted that the fieldworker's worldview is universal—a naive assumption indeed.

2. The problem of order—discerning patterns characteristic of particular actors and events *over time*, as opposed to the order apparent at one moment in time or the order that actors believe to characterize their social practices. Social processes are complex, as are the human beings who engage in them. The consistencies of thought and action that order human practice are not necessarily apparent on the surface, nor are they likely to manifest themselves during a single brief period of observation.

*Insiders' Conscious Models Do Not Necessarily Constitute Reliable Data (Example 1)*

A design team setting out to build a patient education system for migraine sufferers asked a neurologist to provide a realistic sample of the way doctors and patients talk to each other about migraine. Veteran of many years' interaction with migraine patients, the neurologist provided the following dialogue:

Patient:   I'm feeling tired a lot now.
Doctor:   Do you also feel sad or depressed?
P.:   I'm not sure.
D.:   Do you cry often, maybe with no obvious reason?
P.:   No.
D.:   What is your pulse rate?
P.:   56.
A.:   Maybe you'd better take one or two less Inderal per day and see if you feel better.

The design team also contained two anthropologists. Following provision of the sample dialogue above, they carried out extensive observations of interaction between neurologists and migraine patients as well as private interviews with doctors and patients. Their ethnographic fieldnotes contained reports of many conversations between neurologists and migraine patients. Here is a piece of one such conversation:

Doctor:   What are your headaches like? Can you describe one for me?
Patient:   I was about ready to jump [out the window]—the pain. It wasn't a constant pain. . . . I would get like, right back here [patient touches the area below her left ear] it would beat like a heartbeat. I would get like I'm gonna faint. . . . If I've got a cold and am coughing quite often, then I get it.

D.:    Have you ever had headaches before?

P.:    Yeah, I've had headaches . . . maybe once a month or so.

D.:    What was that like?

P.:    [Describes headaches. Doctor decides that these were tension headaches.]

D.:    These headaches now, they're not like that. [Tone of voice indicates that this is a question.]

P.:    . . . I would get, like, after the pain leaves I'd get hot, break out in a sweat, you know? . . . I get roarin' in my ear, and heat . . . [passes hand in front of face, indicating waves of heat over the head.]

D.:    What medicines are you taking?

P.:    [Patient takes a bottle of pills out of her purse and shows it to the doctor.]

D.:    What else do you take?

P.:    He [another doctor] had me on the sprayer [decongestant].

There is a considerable difference between the "realistic" dialogue made up by the physician and this actual dialogue recorded by an anthropologist. Despite the neurologist's expertise, the sample he provided does not constitute good data on the way doctors and patients actually talk to each other. In the expert's model, the interlocutors speak in short, clear messages; in the actual dialogue, the patient's speech is repetitive and rambling. Utterances in the expert's model are unambiguous, whereas some of those in the actual dialogue are more difficult to interpret. For example, it requires some contextual knowledge to understand "He had me on the sprayer." Similarly, the physician asks a question in the form of a declarative statement: "These headaches now, they're not like that." The information-seeking nature of this message is conveyed by the speaker's tone of voice. Messages in the model dialogue are entirely verbal, whereas the real conversation consists of a mixture of verbal and non-verbal messages. In the made-up dialogue, the messages are syntactically much simpler than the real-life utterances. Finally, the questions and answers in the model dialogue are flat—just the facts. In contrast, the actual conversation is quite vivid. The patient uses dramatic imagery to convey the pain of her headaches: "I was about ready to jump [out the window]. . . . "

In short, the expert's reconstruction of a doctor-patient dialogue does not provide a useful model of the real-life process he was trying to characterize. Despite his years of experience in talking with headache patients and his insider status in the world of neurology, his model dialogue is much too simple to be realistic. Reliance on experts' self-reports about their work has long been a standard method of data-gathering for system-building purposes (Forsythe and Buchanan 1989). For reasons made clear by this example, this has led to systems based on simplistic assumptions that have been unable to accommodate the needs of real users in unpredictable situations (ch. 3).

The addition of good ethnography to the design process can help to avoid this problem. Collecting systematic observational data, interviewing a range of practitioners, and addressing disparities between observed and reported phenomena can all help to provide a much more complex and accurate picture of social processes than reliance on experts' conscious models.

### Do-It-Yourself Ethnography in Medical Informatics (Example 2)

Recognition of the contributions of trained fieldworkers to the design process has led to the phenomenon of do-it-yourself ethnography, a trend that anthropologists tend to view with strong reservations. Non-anthropologists do not always understand this reaction. As one reviewer of this paper commented, surely some knowledge of a situation is better than none. The problem is that in ethnography, as in some other pursuits, a little knowledge can be a dangerous thing: superficial social research may confer the illusion of increased understanding when in fact no such understanding has been achieved. This problem is illustrated by the nature of recent do-it-yourself ethnography in medical informatics, in which brief exercises in shadowing, observation, and interviewing have been undertaken from a commonsense stance without engaging the questions that define ethnography as anthropologists understand it. Such an exercise can result in a cognitive hall of mirrors. Without addressing basic issues such as the problem of perspective, researchers have no way of knowing whether they have really understood anything of their informants' worldview or have simply projected and then "discovered" their own assumptions in the data.[2]

What do informaticians do when they set out to do ethnography? The 1995 and 1996 proceedings of the American Medical Informatics Association (AMIA) meetings contain roughly half a dozen papers based on "ethnographic" and "observational" work by researchers who are not social scientists but who have read work by anthropologists and sociologists working in medical informatics (Coble, Maffitt, Orland, and Kahn 1995; Coiera 1996; Rosenal, Forsythe, Musen, and Seiver 1995; Tang, Jaworski, Fellencer, Kreider, LaRosa, and Marquardt 1996; Tang, Jaworski, Fellencer, LaRosa, Lassa, Lipsey, and Marquardt 1995). These studies demonstrate their authors' conception of what qualitative research in general and ethnography in specific entails. The results differ considerably from ethnography as anthropologists understand it.

First, none of these authors appears to have had any serious ethnographic or anthropological training. For example, one senior author has had (as far as I know) no advanced training in either social science or medicine, and learned a method of superficial social scientific inquiry from a weekend workshop conducted by a psychologist. Despite this lack of training and familiarity with anthropological literature, none of the publications expresses reservations about the authors' qualifications or ability to carry out ethnographic research. In short, the authors appear to share an assumption that qualitative research is something anyone can do.

Second, the authors of these papers report short periods of observation, which imply an assumption that what people can be seen to do in a two- or four-hour session is typical of what they do on other occasions. Anthropologists would find the assumption hard to justify and impossible to test with such short-term studies. Use of single observational sessions for each individual also precludes use of some types of triangulation that anthropological fieldworkers find very useful. These include comparing observations of the same individual over time and in different settings; comparing interview and observational data from the same individual, investigating apparent disparities between them; and comparing what people say about each other with what they can be seen to do, again using apparent disparities to guide further investigation. In short, the type of one-shot observation used in these studies implies that seeing and understanding what people are doing is unproblematic, an assumption no anthropologist would share.

The analyses are superficial. In particular, such superficial quasi-ethnography misses the opportunity to make visible and call into question tacit assumptions held by design teams and/or end-users—a characteristic of good ethnographic research that can save both time and money in the process of software development (Forsythe 1995).

TAKING ETHNOGRAPHIC EXPERTISE SERIOUSLY

Anyone with a little knowledge can carry out do-it-yourself social science, just as anyone can write a small program and get it running on a computer. But just as it takes more than a little knowledge to write substantial programs in elegant code, valid social research requires genuine expertise. Yet for some reason, it has been difficult for some technical people to understand that reliable qualitative research requires training and practice.

People in computer science and medical informatics often ask me to suggest "just one article" to enable them to do ethnography themselves. This is absurd. It takes as long to train a competent, Ph.D.-level anthropological fieldworker as it does to train an expert neurosurgeon. Yet who would request the name of a single article on medicine so that he or she could do brain surgery? If nothing else, someone who did so would be subject to stringent legal sanctions, whereas no formal sanctions await those who carry out do-it-yourself ethnographic research. On the contrary, in medical informatics at least, such research is welcomed and is taken at least as seriously as work by experienced social scientists. This too is absurd. If it doesn't make sense to trust medical diagnosis by an amateur in a white coat, why would anyone trust amateur "ethnographic" research by people with no training in social science?

This pattern is particularly puzzling in medical informatics, a field dominated by physicians. Doctors take their own expertise quite seriously; why do they treat ethnography as something that anyone can do? I suggest two reasons. First, educated in a realist tradition and generally given no training in social science, physicians genuinely do not see that ethnographic research requires expertise. As this paper suggests, much of the work required by good ethnography is apparently invisible to them. Second, physicians in the United States occupy a powerful position in society at large as well as in the particular institutions in which they work. Unaccustomed to having their disciplinary assumptions challenged, doctors take for granted that their commonsense beliefs about social phenomena (as expressed, for example, in the "social history" that forms part of the standard history and physical exam) are true and complete. This is presumably one reason for the low rate of user acceptance of some computer systems built for medical settings (Anderson and Aydin 1994). Such systems tend to be based on assumptions about users' needs that are rarely subjected to systematic testing (ch. 1).

DISCUSSION

The misconceptions about ethnographic work that I have described illustrate the fact that people trained in different disciplinary traditions may view the same phenomena in very different ways. The particular conflict in perspectives addressed in this paper has some very real material implications for anthropologists who work in technology development as well as for their supervisors and coworkers from other disciplinary backgrounds. Below I outline some practical consequences that may·result from two issues mentioned above: the apparent invisibility to non-anthropologists of the selectivity and interpretation of the ethnographic data-gathering process, and the fact that the anthropological propensity to identify and question assumptions is not necessarily welcomed in other disciplinary settings.

## *In Which I Am Called a "Walking Tape Recorder"*

Anthropologists who work in interdisciplinary settings sometimes feel that their skills are undervalued by sponsors and colleagues who do not understand what they do. I remember my own chagrin shortly after joining a medical informatics project at hearing the senior physician characterize my role in observing hospital work rounds as being "a walking tape recorder."[3] He did not perceive the creativity of the work I was doing or the fact that another anthropologist would have produced a different narrative.

A corollary of this disparate understanding of fieldwork is a disparate view of the written products of such work. Anthropologists treat field data as intellectual property. One would not normally use another's data without permission, nor would one normally publish from such data without attribution and a possible offer of coauthorship. In contrast, non-anthropologists tend not to see ethnographic field data as intellectual property. On the contrary, consistent with the view of ethnography as something that anyone can do and of fieldworkers themselves as "walking tape recorders," people from science and medicine tend to focus on (quantitative) data analysis while viewing ethnographic data as simply grist for the statistical mill.

This difference in perspective can be a source of conflict. In some projects on which I have worked, physician and computer scientists have wanted to distribute field data that I produced, inviting graduate students and colleagues to conduct and publish their own analyses of the data. One project leader proposed to put hundreds of pages of interview transcripts on the World Wide Web as a sort of public service. (In these cases, the data had been rendered anonymous so that the privacy rights of the individuals studied were not at issue.) Many anthropologists who work in technical settings have encountered some version of this situation, which is typically quite upsetting for the anthropologist. It is distressing to have one's intellectual work overlooked; since ethnographic fieldwork is typically time-consuming, the amount of intellectual work at issue tends to be substantial. In addition, people without social science training may choose to use ethnographic data in ways that strike the fieldworker as invalid or even unethical. The anthropologist involved in this type of conflict may be seen by others as ungenerous or intransigent; in turn, she may see them as exploitative of her and as unconcerned with valid interpretation of the data. What really underlies such conflicts are disparate understandings of the nature and value of ethnographic work and its products.

### Critiquing Colleagues' Assumptions: Biting the Hand     That Feeds Us?

A second example of such disparate understandings concerns the ability of the skilled ethnographer to "see" underlying assumptions. Anthropologists are trained to be reflexive; that is, to attempt to identify and evaluate their own research assumptions as well as those of their respondents. For experienced fieldworkers, it becomes second nature in any situation to listen for what is being taken for granted.

When an anthropologist joins an interdisciplinary design team, it seems natural to apply this ability to the analysis of assumptions held by the team itself as well as those of the formal subjects of ethnographic analysis (such as end-users). In my own experience, this kind of reflexive analysis of design assumptions can be very useful. For example, in the early 1990s, I served as senior anthropologist on a project to build an intelligent patient education system for migraine sufferers. In support of this process, I carried out ethnographic research on neurologists and people with migraine, aided by Myra Brostoff (then a graduate student in anthropology). Attending project meetings, I could not help noticing that the design team was making some assumptions about end-users that did not match what we were seeing during field research. Bringing this disparity to the attention of the designers enabled them to re-think the development plan early in the project, before a great deal of effort had been devoted to developing a prototype that would not have met the user needs we had identified (Forsythe 1995).

As this case demonstrates, the questioning analytical style in which anthropologists are trained can have practical utility in technology design. Not everyone reacts positively to such questioning, however. People from other disciplinary backgrounds and people in positions of authority on design teams may be offended by having their assumptions pointed out, especially when the questioner is someone they view as "non-technical." In some cases, they may not even recognize that they hold particular assumptions quite noticeable to an observer, a manifestation of the not-uncommon problem of "seeing" one's own cultural position.

In addition, in medical informatics, in which physicians are seen as senior to social scientists, the anthropological propensity to name and query tacit assumptions tends to collide with the hierarchical nature of American medicine. This reflects two different views of what it means to question others' assumptions: what anthropologists tend to see as a piece of their ethnographic work may look like insubordination or even betrayal to people trained in other disciplines. As should be obvious, this difference in perspective can create political difficulties for the anthropologist. It may also be awkward for a supervisor who has taken a risk in including an anthropologist on a development team. Even designers who welcome ethnographic insights into users' assumptions and expectations may be less happy when the ethnographic gaze is turned on them. In contrast to the previous example, in which the problem from the anthropologist's point of view is that much of her work is invisible from the standpoint of others, the problem here is the expectation of others that ethnographic work *should* be invisible in a context in which it is not.

## Deleting Ethnographic Work

In my previous ethnographic work on system-building in artificial intelligence and medical informatics (chs. 2, 3), I found that designers consistently discounted those aspects of their own work that involved social interaction or maintenance activities, such as teaching, planning, discussion at meetings, reading and sending email, or backing up their computers. While the people I studied regularly carried out such tasks and often spent a good deal of time on them, they resented having to do so. They dismissed these tasks as "pseudo-work." Such activities were not included when I asked people to describe their work to me. In their accounts, their "real work" was the technical job of system-building, which they saw as restricted to sitting in front of a monitor and writing computer code.

This is an instance of what Leigh Star has called "deletion," a process (often unconscious) in which certain kinds of social phenomena are systematically rendered invisible to those who have reason to know about them. A commonly deleted type of activity is what Star calls "articulation work" (Star 1989: 110). In thinking about their own work processes, technical people tend to delete social (which they think of as "non-technical") work; as I have argued elsewhere, this deletion is carried over into system design as well (chs. 2, 3).

The tendency for social and communicative work to be rendered invisible in technical settings helps to account for the phenomena described in this paper. As I have tried to show, technically trained people may engage in several sorts of deletion in relation to ethnography, which may appear to the naive observer to consist entirely of talking to people. First, when computer scientists and physicians treat ethnography as something that anyone can do, they delete the training, skill, and experience that go into producing good ethnographic work as well as the analytical process it entails. Several specific examples of deleted ethnographic work were described in the list of misconceptions offered above. Second, as I illustrated with examples from medical informatics, when non-anthropologists borrow ethnography, they tend to delete the accompanying philosophical stance and to treat it as a decontextualized bundle of data-gathering techniques. This defeats the purpose and much of the power of the ethnographic approach. And third, when people take offense at having their own design assumptions identified, they overlook the fact that all of us take things for granted that may affect our work. Uncovering tacit orthodoxies is precisely what ethnography is supposed to do. In other words, not only is ethnography not "just a matter of common sense," part of its purpose is to identify our common sense—and to help us to assess it.

# CHAPTER ELEVEN

# Disappearing Women in the Social World of Computing

Scientists' accounts of their work typically stress the objectivity and gender neutrality of their practice.[1] However, a feminist perspective reveals much in such practice that is highly gendered. Both female bodies and experience tend to be treated as inherently anomalous in the male world of high technology. Drawing upon ethnographic data from long-term participant observation in the overlapping worlds of artificial intelligence (AI) and medical informatics, this paper undertakes to examine the ways in which both females and femaleness are constructed as problematic in day-to-day work settings, analyzing the social and cultural work used to manage female "Otherness."

The deletion of women is one of many patterns of selectivity that characterize daily practice in AI and medical informatics. For convenience, I will use the latter term to refer to my research domain at the intersection of these two fields. My ethnographic material is the outcome of eight years' full-time participant observation in five laboratories, four in academia and one in business (chs. 1–3). I present the material under the device of "the Lab" in order to protect the privacy of individuals (particularly the small number of women in these settings).

Medical informatics is the application of intelligent systems technology from computer science to problems in medicine. The work of medical informatics is to build intelligent computer systems to support medical practice (Buchanan and Shortliffe 1984).[2] As a participant-observer, this strikes me as a very male-oriented field, a view reinforced by the comments and experiences of women who work in it. In this paper, I attempt to explore what this male orientation means and how it is expressed in day-to-day practice. I will pay particular attention to the ways in which apparently unrelated aspects of the disciplinary "culture" work together to render women and their work less visible.

## BACKGROUND ON MEDICAL INFORMATICS

Men and women in the workplace encounter each other in the context of particular disciplinary cultures as well as work environments shaped in part by the proportion of men and women who work in a given field. This section provides some background on medical informatics with respect to both factors: the ideal of scientific neutrality and the low representation of women in medical informatics and in computer science as a whole.

### Ideology of Science as Neutral

Contemporary anthropologists tend to portray science and technology as inherently cultural. This leads to an interest in the meanings that scientists bring to their practice (chs. 2, 3; Hess and Layne 1992; Traweek 1988a) and in locating actors and technology in relation to each other and to broader political contexts (Hess 1995; Latour 1987; Suchman 1994; Traweek 1992). In contrast, researchers in medical informatics approach their work as positivists. They see science as the pursuit of objective truth and understand truth as culturally neutral. Their attitude is that while scientists may be cultural, science itself is not.

As the following exchange illustrates, this attitude is applied explicitly to the notion of gender. The exchange took place after a Lab meeting at which I mentioned the idea of writing this paper:

*Lab head*: "Science is supposed to be about ideas."
*DEF*: "Some of the most powerful ideas in our culture are about gender."
*Lab head*: "Yes, but that's for social scientists. . . . The study of gender issues is for social scientists. The study of computer science issues is for computer scientists. . . . I'm trying to separate the people who do science from the ideas they investigate" (January 24, 1994).

Interpretive anthropologists make a careful distinction between shared ideals and practice as it works out "on the ground" (Geertz 1973, 1983). In contrast, unless experience leads them to notice a disparity, people in medical informatics tend to assume that ideals and practice are congruent (ch. 2). Perhaps because their field inherits the cognitive bias of AI and cognitive science (Suchman 1990; Woolgar 1987), these scientists do not systematically compare normative description with observable action. Like the laboratory head quoted above, both men and women in medical informatics assert that science is gender neutral. As an anthropologist, I translate that to mean that science as it *should* be practiced is gender neutral.

Whereas most men in medical informatics appear to assume that their everyday life in the Lab reflects this ideal, some women point out that this is not the case. They complain of sexism in their own work settings, in the funding of research, and in the operation of professional organizations within the field. My own observation is that medical informatics as practiced is not at all neutral with respect to gender: the default assumptions in both everyday interaction and in system design often reflect the perspectives and life experience of men.[3] Thus, what men in this field perceive as neutral, many women perceive as male-dominated. Despite the ideology of scientific neutrality, then, women, their work, and the qualities attributed to them are marked in these settings. In relation to what Haraway calls "the unmarked masculine" (Haraway 1989: 357), women's work, life experience, and bodies appear as "inherently anomalous" (Lock and Gordon 1988: 345)—if indeed they are seen at all.

## Small Numbers of Women

In demographic terms, women *are* anomalous in medical informatics, as they are in computer science generally.[4] The normative path to a faculty or research career in computer science is through a Ph.D. in computer science or a subdiscipline such as AI. In 1992, women earned only 12 percent of the U.S. doctorates awarded in computer science (Gries and Marsh 1992). According to a 1990 National Science Foundation report (1990), women constituted 8 percent of computer science faculty overall, but only 4 percent of full professors.

The small proportion of women in computer science has received a good deal of attention within the discipline, particularly in AI, which (in the context of computer science) has an unusually large number of women (Female Graduate Students 1983; Pearl, Pollack, Riskin, Thomas, Wolf, and Wu 1990). In the late 1980s, the American Association for Artificial Intelligence (AAAI), the main professional body in AI, convened a committee to encourage women and minorities to work in the field. This committee drafted a series of suggestions. Reflecting the assumption that science is neutral, all of them were directed toward students and young people who were yet to choose a career direction. None of the suggestions addressed working conditions within the discipline or considered the possibility that the work itself might be seen by women or minorities as biased (unpublished draft memo of July 18, 1987).

Medical informatics is also a largely male field. The standard career path is through an M.D. followed by several years of training in one of the dozen postdoctoral training programs funded by the National Library of Medicine (NLM), an institute of National Institutes of Health. In contrast to computer science, there seem to be no formal efforts in medical informatics to track representation by gender. When I contacted the NLM to inquire about the proportion of men and women in their traineeships, they said that they did not keep statistics by gender or race. However, we can gain some notion of the proportion of women among established members of the field by examining the list of fellows elected by the American College of Medical Informatics (ACMI), the professional body that constitutes the "old boys" in medical informatics.[5] One hundred forty-eight people were elected by ACMI as fellows between 1984 and 1992. Of these, 130 (88 percent) were male and 18 (12 percent) were female (American College of Medical Informatics 1994).

The normative qualification for faculty status in medical informatics is an M.D. and a Ph.D. Of these degrees, the M.D. is seen as far more important. Major male players within the field hold an M.D. and Ph.D. or an M.D. alone. A few hold a Ph.D. alone, but their professional credibility is reduced by the lack of a medical degree. Because of the importance accorded the latter, quite a few men in the field first obtain a Ph.D. in computer science or medical information science, and then attend medical school without doing an internship or residency. Since these individuals never practice clinically, the main purpose of their medical training seems to be the political goal of acquiring credibility in medical informatics by obtaining the M.D. They also acquire some knowledge of medicine but very little knowledge of clinical practice.

In relation to this normative model for entrance into medical informatics, it is worth noting that it is a career path followed mainly by men. Of the eighteen female ACMI fellows as of 1992, only three hold the M.D./Ph.D., and one holds an M.D. alone. Most of the remaining women appear to hold qualifications in library science, nursing, or education.[6] The pattern suggested by these figures applies to the field in general: while the proportion of women entering medicine has risen dramatically over the past several decades, very few female physicians go into medical informatics. Instead, most women enter this field by way of nursing or medical library science.

In sum, women are a small minority of professionals in computer science and medical informatics. In the lab settings in which I have carried out field-work, the proportion of female researchers is well below the 15 percent identified as the "critical mass" for women in science (Dresselhaus, Franz, and Clark 1994: 1392; Etzkowitz, Kemelgor, Neuschatz, Uzzi, and Alonzo 1994: 51). One of the laboratories had no female scientists at all. In contrast, the secretarial and administrative support staff was entirely female.

## MY RELATION TO THE TOPIC OF THIS PAPER

In postmodernism we have come to understand the importance of viewing individuals—ethnographers as well as informants—as positioned (Behar 1993; Linden 1993; Rosaldo 1993). Trying to "see" and write about the cultural work of deleting women has led me to try to locate myself in relation to the computing worlds I study and the family in which I grew up. In attempting this task, I am grateful for the example of other social scientists who have written themselves into their stories (Behar 1993; Haraway 1989, 1991; Linden 1993; Polanyi 1995; Rapp 1993; Rosaldo 1993; Traweek 1988a, 1992).

I am the daughter of two pioneering computer scientists—a much-honored man whose name is still well known two decades after his death, and a visionary woman who received relatively little professional recognition during her lifetime and whose career has been largely erased since her death in 1980. As the product of their union, I have contradictory feelings about computer science that reflect their respective positions within and without the establishment of academic computer science.

The devaluation of women in science and computing influenced me powerfully as a teenager and young adult, as I watched my mother struggle to negotiate her own career. Her frustration and suppressed anger at the barriers she encountered were very clear to me. In trying to establish my own identity as a woman and a social scientist in the professional worlds of computing and medicine, I have reconnected with my mother's struggle, although she died before I began this study. My concern with the boundary between AI and anthropology has provided a forum for negotiating my own professional identity, working out the relationship between my parents' work and mine, and between the disparate worldviews embodied in our respective disciplines. The theme of this paper brings these worlds together. In one way, then, the paper is about what I observed and experienced in the field. In another, it is about what happened to my mother in computer science, which helped to shape who I am and what I saw in the field.

## Disappearing My Mother

Imagine two bright people; let's call them George and Sandra. In the late 1930s, they graduated from Swarthmore College and went to Brown University to do graduate work in mathematics. George encountered supportive faculty and finished his Ph.D. in four years. Sandra, in contrast, found that her advisor did not approve of female mathematicians. She eventually left Brown and completed a master's degree in mathematics at Smith. In 1941, on the day George finished his Ph.D., he and Sandra married. George went into the military and taught meteorology. After the war, George worked for a research institute and then obtained a faculty position in meteorology at UCLA, from which he moved into mathematics. Sandra worked for a while in industry, but by the late 1940s was at home full-time, caring for the couple's two young children.

Cut to the late 1960s. George is now a full professor at a major university on the West Coast. An applied mathematician, he is helping to develop the new field of computer science and has become internationally known. He has just attained his goal of persuading the university to start a new computer science department, of which he is to be chair. In this position, he assembles a computer science faculty, which by the way contains no women. (In the succeeding 25 years, this department produces female Ph.D.'s but hires very few and does not tenure one until 1995 or 1996.) Sandra has also become a computer scientist, although without an academic base. She would like a position at the university but the nepotism rule works against her. So she turns to secondary education and teaches high school mathematics. There she accomplishes what George did in the university: she fights for and eventually succeeds in introducing a computer science curriculum, one of the first in the country. She is also a prolific author.

Cut now to the 1990s. George died in 1972, in his fifties. At the university, his name is omnipresent: a building is named after him, a widely used campus computer bears his name, and the department holds an annual lectureship in his memory. Sandra also died relatively young, in 1980, but where is her name? No building or computer is named after her (although the department did add her name to George's lectureship after her death, perpetuating her memory as faculty spouse). George continues to be honored as a pioneer of computer science—but Sandra was a pioneer as well. With little in the way of institutional support and none at all from the university, she wrote or co-authored seven books in computer science, including the first textbook in the field. That text was translated into several languages and went into a second edition. Two decades later, some of her work is still in print, but her name seems to have vanished.

> A professor is putting together an encyclopedia of computer science. He puts a notice on Systers, an email network of women, requesting information on female candidates for inclusion in this volume. I send him a message about my mother, offering to assemble a biographical statement on her. Seeing the name Forsythe, he writes back excitedly to ask me to update the entry he already has for my father. The notion of an entry on my mother has disappeared.

As a story about the lives of men and women in science, this one is not unusual (see Keller 1977, 1983; McGrayne 1993). Some of my mother's women friends had similar experiences; some of them were worse. Perhaps you have a similar story. Or perhaps you imagine that things these days are quite different.

I have told you something about my relationship to the subject matter of this paper. This should be enough to dispel any illusion that mine is a neutral voice. But whose voice is ever neutral? Having conveyed something of the background from which I see and interpret the experiences of women in science, I now turn back to describing what I saw in the Lab. The next section addresses the question, What is it like to be a woman in the Lab?

THE LAB AS "MALE TERRITORY"

The starting point for this investigation was my gradual realization that in medical informatics, women are second-class citizens. They—we—simply "don't count" (see below) the way men do. While the construction of women as "Other" is of course not restricted to this field, beliefs and expectations may be put into practice quite differently in different contexts of action. I will illustrate some ways in which notions of female Otherness are expressed in the course of day-to-day life in the Lab.

To make it through to post-doctoral or faculty status, women must be capable of interacting successfully as "one of the boys." In addition to having good technical skills, this requires them to be bright, tough, and assertive. To get along with their male colleagues (which does not imply equality), women must be able to withstand teasing, testing, and sometimes outright harassment. I will give two examples. Appropriate to the technology-centered setting, they involve the use of computers to convey representations of female bodies or bodily experience.

The first example concerns a screen saver. All of the Lab computers have screen saver programs that come on to save power if a machine is out of use for more than a few minutes. One day some male graduate students installed on a large-screened machine a screen saver that flashed a series of giant images of scantily clad women in seductive poses. There were no parallel images of men. Since the machine was located in the Lab's open-plan central work area, these images were visible to everyone who walked through. As far as I know, no Lab member beside me expressed objections to the new screen saver. Since I thought it a bad idea, I talked with one of the grad students responsible for installing it. He found the situation funny. This man jokes a lot with women about gender and clearly enjoys getting a rise out of them. When asked why, he replied:

> Because I think an awful lot of women are way too serious about gender and you can't have a rational discussion about gender with them. They just won't change their minds (January 24, 1994).

Eventually I brought up the matter with the Lab head, pointing out that I thought the screen saver created an uncomfortable climate for women. That argument didn't seem to carry much weight. Then I pointed out that some of his female graduate students were foreign and came from countries with more conservative notions of propriety than ours. The idea that foreign women might be shocked by the screen saver seemed to carry more weight than the sensibilities of women in general. The head of the Lab asked the students to remove the screen saver.

Installation of the screen saver was directed toward women as a class rather than toward any one individual. In contrast, a second incident targeted a particular graduate student. One day shortly after her arrival in the Lab, she found a new file icon in her folder on the desktop of her Macintosh. Out of curiosity she clicked on the new icon, which started a sound clip of the orgasm scene from the movie "When Harry Met Sally." The clip produced loud, sexual noises and apparently could not be stopped. While it was running, another female graduate student came in, one of the foreign students mentioned above. Both women stared at the screen, appalled. They did not discuss this incident with each other, nor did they tell any senior Lab member about the incident. A year or so later, when I learned about it, I asked one of the students why she hadn't mentioned it. She replied: "I guess it just comes with the territory. I mean, this *is* male territory. It's a computer science department."

While writing this paper, I emailed an informant from the Lab to ask about this incident. Assuring him that I didn't want to know who had done the deed, I inquired whether it might have been intended as harassment, teasing, or flirting. He replied as follows:

> A certain party . . . discovered the "When Harry Met Sally" Big O sound clip for the Mac somewhere on the net, and downloaded it to the machine in the lab. . . . This person said to me, "Hey, click on this icon," or something like that, to get me to invoke the sound bite . . . and I did, and it was funny. Some-time along the line [the female grad student] was coming in to work, and by default that [machine] was her workstation, so the prankster decided to name the file that invoked the sound bite "[her name]," so that she'd click on it. Everyone sort of scattered; [she] took the bait and was embarrassed by it (which was the point of the joke, in my opinion). My feeling is that there was absolutely no intention of harassment. Neither was the intention to flirt. It was a practical joke played by someone who was not known for his sensitivity to issues of so-called "sexual harassment." I believe the joke would have been played on whomever would be the next person to sit at the computer, and [she] was the lucky one.

Where I and the recipient are inclined to interpret this incident as sexual harassment, this man sees a harmless practical joke. If nothing else, this demonstrates the considerable difference in perspective that may separate male and female co-workers within one laboratory. Women who work in computer-related settings are likely to be confronted from time to time with similar "jokes." These help to create a climate that women tend to interpret as hostile. As one woman in the Lab put it, speaking about the second incident above, "These guys are such jerks. This is what we have to put up with around here."

## BRACKETING OUT WOMEN

The deletion of women is not a uniform or straightforward phenomenon; it is the outcome of ongoing cultural work of varying subtlety that occurs in a wide range of contexts. For example:

> I am working with a senior physician to develop a category set of "medical information sources." After he has listed as information sources doctors, literature, computer databases, family members of patients, and "the community," I finally inquire, "What about nurses?" He replies, "Nurses don't count."

Researchers in medical informatics make assumptions about which people and types of people "count." Usually these notions remain tacit, but from time to time they become explicit. In multiple ways, through the most everyday comments and gestures, men are defined as belonging to this category and women are bracketed out of it. Such comments add up. They help to marginalize women by framing them or their work as unimportant or unsatisfactory and rendering them less visible in the eyes of their male—and sometimes female—colleagues.

Various biases or strategies operate in the Lab environment to bracket women out. I'm not sure what terms to use here: "strategy" implies intentionality, which is not always easy to ascertain; "bias" implies the possibility of neutrality or objectivity, which I do not believe. What I present below are my own inferences, based on watching and talking with people over time, about a piece of the tacit logic in their shared words and actions. While the consequences of these patterns are not necessarily known to or intended by everyone who contributes to them, they help to create different work climates for men and women. This disparity tends to empower men and disempower women.

Below I describe two major ways in which women are rendered invisible in medical informatics. The first involves the deletion of people who perform certain types of work. The second is the widespread practice of defining even senior women in relation to men, whereas men are defined in terms of their own work.

## Discounting Certain Types of Work(ers)

Some women in the workplace are rendered invisible through the systematic bracketing out of people who perform work that is gendered as female. (In contrast, those who do work that is gendered as male—e.g., physicians—are not overlooked.) Whether the more fundamental bias is against the nature of the work in question (see below) or against the fact that this work is performed by women is difficult to say. The work categories I will consider are first, administrators and secretaries, and second, nurses and librarians.

### Overlooking Clerical Support Staff

I walk into a lab that I have been told has no women. The first thing I see are two women—an administrator and a secretary, both seated at desks in the central reception area. Over the next two years, as I go in and out of this laboratory, I learn that the administrator has worked at the university for decades and is acknowledged as the local expert on university procedure and the federal funding agency that supports the lab. A no-nonsense person, she speaks her mind to students and the Lab head alike. The younger secretary is acquiring the same style.

No one could miss these women's presence in the lab, and their work is clearly essential to its functioning. What does it mean to say that the laboratory in which they work consists only of men?

In all of the laboratories in which I worked, research rested upon the support work of administrators and secretaries. These people are in the laboratory every weekday, interact with researchers on a social basis, and are invariably female. Although an unquestioned part of each medical informatics workplace, they are not considered to be "in" medical informatics and do not count as "Lab members." Lab members are researchers: faculty, postdocs, research associates, and graduate students (but not undergraduates).

In claiming that support staff are overlooked, I do not mean to suggest that they or their work are not seen as essential. On the contrary, what they do is universally acknowledged as necessary; among other things, proposals would never go out the door without their help. However, their work is not defined as *important*. This usage reflects Lab members' highly selective notion of what counts as "real work." As I describe elsewhere (ch. 2), my informants consistently discount those aspects of their own work that involve social interaction or maintenance, such as teaching, planning, discussion at meetings, reading and sending email, or backing up their computers. While everyone has to do such tasks, they are resented and dismissed as "pseudo-work." In this world, the "important work" is the decontextualized, technical job of system-building: sitting in front of a monitor and writing computer code. In bracketing out those whose tasks largely involve what Star calls "articulation work" (Star 1989: 110), Lab members replicate this restriction of "real work" to a very narrow, formal band of activities.

### Discounting Nurses and Librarians

The first category of discounted workers mentioned above was clerical support staff, who do not do research. A second discounted category involves people who do carry out research in medical informatics and are thus eligible to be Lab members.

Medical informatics draws researchers from several fields; these fields are gendered. Almost all the physicians and computer scientists in medical informatics are male; researchers with backgrounds in nursing and library science are almost entirely female. While the work of medical informatics is interdisciplinary, the normative values of the field reflect those of institutionalized medicine. Thus, when women move from nursing or library science into research careers in medical informatics, they encounter two kinds of bias: the tendency to discount women, and the low status accorded nurses and medical librarians in relation to physicians. In addition to their practice-based training, which is not viewed with great respect by physicians, some nurses and librarians also hold academic Ph.D.'s. This increases their prestige but only to an extent limited by a third bias characteristic of medical informatics (and medicine): the low value accorded the Ph.D. in relation to the M.D. These disciplinary assumptions serve to marginalize women and may even be treated be as stigmatizing (Goffman 1963).

Two examples will illustrate this. Both reflect the experience of a nurse who also holds a Ph.D. in a technical field and has been extremely productive for years as an academic informatics researcher. One day this woman was scheduled to give a talk in medical informatics at another university where she was well known. The flyer posted to announce the talk listed the speaker's R.N. but not her Ph.D. I see two meanings in this omission. First, it illustrates the relative lack of importance accorded the Ph.D. in relation to the M.D. The former was treated as disposable, whereas the names of physicians rarely appear in professional contexts without the M.D. Second, the retention of the speaker's R.N. on the announcement reflects the viewpoint that "once a nurse, always a nurse." It is in this sense that nursing qualification can be seen as stigmatizing in this field. No matter how many other degrees she obtains, how many papers she publishes, or what seniority she achieves, to the physicians in medical informatics this woman is a nurse. As we saw above, in medical informatics, "nurses don't count!"

In the second example, this same researcher was invited to participate in a public panel to discuss developments in nursing informatics. She arrived at the podium and encountered her fellow panelists. They were three "old boys", all physicians—an interesting choice of discussants on the concept of nursing informatics. The following dialogue took place:

*Old boy*:    I thought there were going to be four doctors here [on the panel].
*Woman*:    There are.
*Old boy*:    Who's the fourth?

*Woman*:    Me!

*Old boy*:    I didn't know you were a physician.

In medical informatics, as in American medicine generally, the doctorate in philosophy is not seen as conferring the right to use the title "doctor." As many Ph.D.'s working in the field have discovered, to call oneself "Dr." is to risk the accusation of misrepresenting oneself as a "real" doctor, that is, a physician.

## Assimilating Women to the World of Men

I have argued that a frequent strategy for disappearing women is to bracket them out by discounting their work. Another is to assimilate them to the world of men. In the most egregious version of this phenomenon, women are assumed to *be* men. I encountered a striking face-to-face example of such assimilation:

> One day outside the Lab I meet the only female faculty member in computer science at a certain university. She calls herself a feminist, and like my mother, she specializes in programming languages. Seeking common ground, I ask her if she is familiar with the work of my mother, Alexandra Forsythe. She says, "I thought that was a man!"

Men are not the only ones to disappear women.

It is normal in medical informatics to define female researchers in relation to men. Even full professors are described in this way—if they are women. However, male researchers past the doctorate are not often defined by their relation to men or women. This relational approach to the construction of female scientists is not thought of as strange or degrading, except by some of the women so described; it is certainly not intended as a joke.

I first encountered this practice when I moved with the Lab to a new university. The head of the Lab returned from a meeting, laughing that the department chair had referred to me as "your girl." Thereafter, we both noticed the frequency with which I was framed in medical informatics settings as "his girl." Indeed, I quickly learned to define myself in this way as a defense against wholesale deletion. Faced with an "old boy" staring blankly at me as I tried to engage him in conversation, I learned to say, "I work in Steve's lab."[7] If the person chose to recognize my existence and had read any of my papers, the unapologetic response would have been, "Oh, you're Steve's anthropologist!"

Whereas women are defined relationally, men are defined in terms of what they do. This disparity is one reflection of a whole set of different expectations about male and female researchers and male and female careers. Many of the expectations applied to women are familiar (and sexist) carry-overs from the wider society. Insofar as they are not applied to men, they change the options open to male and female scientists, reducing the choices available to women and imposing costs should they choose to defy these expectations. What is expected of women promotes their disappearance into the shadow of men.

Male graduate students are trained to go out in the world and pursue their own interests. If they are bright and have behaved decently during their training, they can expect to remain in the network of their sponsor(s) throughout their career. In medical informatics, a great deal is decided by and through the "old boys'" network. The support of an influential mentor helps researchers to obtain information, employment, funding, and guidance.

In contrast, female students and young faculty are not always encouraged to go out and pursue their own interests, nor are they as likely to remain in a protective network if and when they leave. Instead, women are sometimes pressured to pursue their mentor's interests rather than their own. For example, I observed a female assistant professor constrained by her laboratory head to put his name on a major proposal that she had written. In a soft money lab, everyone works at the pleasure of the chief; this renders even research faculty very vulnerable. This woman capitulated to her boss's threat that to refuse was to put her career at risk. In another laboratory, another female soft money researcher was pressured by her laboratory head to name a senior male as an author on a paper to which he had contributed nothing. When she resisted, her mentor accused her of being "ungenerous." Feeling threatened, she also capitulated. Finally, in a third laboratory, a third female soft money researcher refused to give in to the demands of her laboratory head in another dispute over a question of authorship. Afterward, this man described her to me repeatedly as selfish, although her argument as he recounted it seemed reasonable to me. Since then this woman has been refused a promotion and has encountered difficulties in obtaining funding. Whether there is any connection between these setbacks and her defiance of an "old boy," I don't know.

Female researchers are caught in a double bind. They need a mentor to get anywhere. Since senior figures in this field are almost entirely male, mentors are almost certainly men. To remain in a mentor's good graces, a woman must be useful to him—which generally means producing publications with his name on them. However, given the practice of defining women in relation to men, a woman collaborating with a senior male is likely to get lost in his shadow. This makes it difficult for a woman to acquire a reputation as an independent researcher. Unlike men, women are not expected to "grow up" and develop into laboratory heads. After watching a number of women caught in this situation, I have come to think of the role they play as "wife at work." In some cases, these women have a warm personal relationship with the sponsor, to whom they are bound with ties of mutual dependence. In other cases, the relationship looks exploitative or even abusive.

To make matters worse, laboratory heads will hire a male researcher away from a different laboratory, but "old boys" seem reluctant to hire away women. Is this seen as stealing another man's "girl"? Or perhaps they are just reluctant to hire women. In any case, female researchers may find themselves caught out of sight in their mentor's shadow, having few options and little alternative to an unequal relationship in which the mentor holds most of the cards.

## Disappearing the Female Body

I have described several beliefs and practices that work to disappear women in computer-related work settings. However, despite these patterns, some women under some circumstances manage to carry on and even prosper. In contrast to nurses and librarians in medical informatics, female computer scientists are not easily bracketed out by male colleagues based on the nature of their work. Bright women who do research perceived as "hard" and who are capable of functioning as "one of the boys" are (within limits) accorded the status of honorary men. However, life events may expose the fictive nature of this device, facing men with the challenge of dealing with problematic female bodies and experiences.[8] Once when I observed this, the solution chosen was to disappear the female body.

> I walk into the office one afternoon and see John, a Lab researcher, peering at a computer monitor with Susan, a researcher from one of the Lab's industrial affiliates. They collaborate for the most part over the Internet, and Susan hasn't visited the Lab for many months. It is clear at a glance that she is pregnant, so I ask her when the baby is due. Later, after Susan has gone home, John tells me he is glad that I inquired about her baby. He had noticed that she looked

larger than usual, but didn't want to say anything in case she had simply gained a lot of weight recently. He said, "A male friend comes by and looks fat, you could pat him in the belly and tell him. But a woman, you can't do that, you never know what might happen" (January 24, 1994).

John worked all day with Susan, his colleague of several years, and never said a word about her pregnancy. One might interpret this simply as shyness, but John is not noticeably shy. Instead, I suggest that Susan's visibly pregnant body presented him with a problem. In the male territory of the Lab, Susan gets along well as one of the boys, but this reframing is difficult to maintain in the face of her protruding belly—dramatic testimony that she is not in fact a boy at all. Unsure how to deal with that dangerous and unpredictable belly, John simply deletes it. Having made Susan's anomalous female body disappear, he carries on working with her all day as "one of the boys," worried only by a slight suspicion that perhaps he should have said something after all.

DISCUSSION

I have presented some information on a disciplinary culture and its expression in the context of local scientific practice that (male) practitioners describe as gender neutral and I as a feminist see as highly gendered. My goal is to understand this difference in perspective. I have tried to show that despite the ideology of scientific neutrality, medical informatics as practiced is both demographically and politically male. If one counts secretaries, administrators, and students as well as female researchers, the work settings I have been describing contain quite a few women. Yet the Lab strikes men and women alike as "male territory." This impression results in part from the marginalization of women, their work, and their bodies, leaving men in symbolic possession of the Laboratory core. In this field, a male scientist is seen as a scientist; a female scientist is seen as a woman (see Tavris 1992: 16–21, 335n.5, quoting Minnich 1990: 79).

The deletion of certain gendered categories of work is translated in the course of daily practice into the deletion of certain categories of workers. As we have seen, the work of secretarial and administrative workers, nurses, and medical librarians is in various ways overlooked or devalued. In addition, the tendency to define women in terms of men and the differing expectations for career development of men and women push women into the shadow of male supervisors and collaborators. In a field in which so much work is collaborative, women often face a double bind: if they cooperate, they may be exploited and/or disappear altogether; if they don't, they are accused of being uncollegial.

To moderate this dismal picture, I will add two caveats. First, while the discounting of maintenance and articulation work in medical informatics promotes the deletion of women, not everyone rendered invisible in this way is female. A small minority of nurses and medical librarians are men. Within medicine itself, men as well as women who adopt less prestigious specialties (e.g., pediatrics or family medicine as opposed to surgery) are to a certain extent bracketed out by other physicians. More significantly, other, non-clerical types of support work may render individuals of both sexes invisible. Barley has described the work of technicians in a range of practice settings, including medicine (Barley 1986, 1994; Barley and Bechky 1994). He argues that technicians' essential contribution to scientific work is routinely overlooked both by the scientists they support and by social scientists who investigate laboratory life. In the settings described in this paper, the (mostly male) computer programmers and computer systems administrators may well receive treatment somewhat comparable to that accorded the technicians described by Barley. This is an issue I would like to pursue.

Second, it is important to acknowledge that secretaries, administrators, nurses, and librarians are actors as well as acted upon. While their male/senior co-workers may bracket them out, they themselves are capable of deleting other individuals, including men. For example, during a job search for a part-time secretarial position in the Lab, the most highly qualified individual (on paper at least) was a man. However, the notion of a male secretary in that time and place was extremely unusual. The impressive resume simply disappeared—not (as far as I know) because of objections from the senior scientist in the Lab, who had the official say in the matter, but rather because the secretarial staff just couldn't see a man performing "women's work."

## Implications for Change

What does the material in this paper imply about policies and programs that might affect the representation and experience of women in computing worlds? Public efforts to increase the proportion of women in computer science generally treat the problem as a "pipeline issue." That is, they assume that the problem will be solved (or at least ameliorated) if more women can be encouraged to go into computer science. Consequently, such efforts focus on programs to encourage girls and young women to study science and to consider technical careers. While any attention devoted to encouraging female scholarship is probably a good idea, the pipeline model is based on the questionable assumption that if women can be induced to go into computer fields, they will stay there. This ignores the fact that there are already women in these fields and that they and their work are often subject to unequal treatment. Many women (including my mother) have already tried very hard to have careers in computer science; not all have found their efforts rewarded. I suggest that if efforts to change this state of affairs are to be successful, they should take a proactive approach to issues of retention and promotion within the field, as well as encourage women to enter it.

## Why Aren't More Female Computer Scientists Feminists?

Given the ethnographic material I have presented, one might wonder why more women in computer science aren't overt feminists.[9] During my own fieldwork, I encountered numerous women who asserted that gender was not an issue in their own work lives; some who cautiously mentioned gender as a possible issue for their own personal careers, but did not express common cause with other women in the field or appear to consider engaging in collective action; and a very small number of conscious feminists. In dealing with female graduate students who asserted that gender was irrelevant to them, I often wondered whether to try to make it visible to them or to leave them in the more comfortable (and, to my mind, mistaken) belief that "all that" was taken care of decades ago. Feminists tend to be highly aware of gender as a social variable. I suggest that at least some women inclined to "see" gender-related patterns may find computer worlds too uncomfortable to work in. (There are a few software companies headed by women, and a few computer science departments with more than token numbers of women. This is not the norm, however.) Adding to this the hostility that I at least encountered from some computer scientists in response to this paper (see below), I suspect that women who overtly question gender-related patterns from a less than senior position may have to deal with considerable reaction. I speculate that the prevailing tacit deletion of women and gender issues, plus the gendered power hierarchy in computer fields, may combine to pressure women either to join in the silence or to leave the field.[10] It would be interesting to carry out "exit interviews" with women who leave computer science and medical informatics beyond the Ph.D. in order to assess whether perceived discrimination against women is mentioned as a factor in their decisions.

## How Have People Reacted to This Paper?

In order to see how people in computer science and medical informatics would respond to what I have written about gender issues in the worlds of computer science and medical informatics, I have given copies of this paper to men and women in both computer-related fields and in social science. Their responses to the paper have been interesting. Feminist women in both social science and computer science have been enthusiastic about the paper. One female computer scientist said, "Everything you wrote about in your paper has happened to me." A nurse/Ph.D. in informatics read the paper, liked it, and offered more stories to confirm what I had written. On the other hand, a non-ideological female computer scientist who has nevertheless been active on behalf of women in her field asked to read the paper but has not responded to several requests for feedback on it. I have no idea what she thought of it.

Of the men to whom I gave the paper, two male social scientists reacted quite negatively. One untenured man told me with considerable emotion that the things I describe happen to men as well and that they have nothing to do with gender. Another, more senior, said that the paper was simply about me and that he "had nothing to say about it." A male engineer said, "Aren't you just trying to defend your mother?" I am not sure why he thought she might require my defense. A male Ph.D. in medical informatics explained to me in fatherly fashion that the paper is purely anecdotal and that I should rewrite it with facts if I want people in his field to take it seriously. Several other men in computer science and medical informatics have received one or more copies of the paper with requests for critique, but never seem to remember having received it when I ask for feedback. One of these men has received considerable attention for his expressed interest in fostering women in the field. When I asked him about the paper face to face, he looked angry and simply turned away.

It seems that many men and some women find the topic of this paper uncomfortable and would prefer not to address it. Bracketing things out through silence is of course a major strategy of deletion, precisely what the paper is about. To attempt to break that silence is to risk eliciting a surprising amount of hostility, suggesting that to some people, at least, naming a pattern of deletion is a greater wrong than the deletion itself. As Traweek notes,

> We do engender the production of knowledge everywhere and we do not like to think about it. Our silence is a compelling silence, muffled by laughter, anger, and the shock of recognition (Traweek 1988b: 252).

CONCLUSION

I want to conclude by referring to an apparently paradoxical aspect of the social and cultural work used to manage female "Otherness" in medical informatics. I have argued that by discounting their work and systematically bracketing them out of the category of "people who count," professionals in medical informatics marginalize women. In the sense that it renders them less visible to their peers and perhaps to themselves as well, such cultural work makes women disappear.

At the same time, I have pointed out that women are subject to a good deal of teasing and testing, which some men see as joking and some women see as harassment. In apparent contrast to the first trend, this treatment renders women hyper-visible, constantly recreating and commenting upon their condition as marked.

The paradox, I think, is real: women in the settings I have described do get jerked back and forth between being constructed as invisible and as all too visible, an experience I imagine myself to have shared as an anomalous observing participant. What they are rarely allowed is something their male colleagues take for granted: the experience of being visible if they wish, invisible if they choose, and in any case simply accepted as normal scientists.

# CHAPTER TWELVE

# George and Sandra's Daughter, Robert's Girl: Doing Ethnographic Research in My Parents' Field

Whom are we studying when we do fieldwork?[1] Whose life is chronicled in our ethnographic texts? Familiar as these questions have become in anthropological circles (Behar 1993: 267–342; Behar and Gordon 1995; Geertz 1988; Okely and Callaway 1992), they take on new dimensions for those of us positioned as what Deborah Heath calls "science kin." If ethnography and autobiography are "entangled" for all anthropologists, as Visweswaran argues in *Fictions of Feminist Ethnography* (1994: 6), they became thoroughly enmeshed when I set out to investigate my parents' field of computer science.

While some authors seek ways to write themselves into their ethnographic texts, I struggle here with the opposite problem: gaining enough distance from my location to write about it at all. I have written numerous analytical papers about this research, papers in which I am present as an intellectual voice. Compared to these papers, the two in which I have tried to address the personal meaning of this work have been extremely difficult to write.[2]

The dichotomous categories we use to describe and teach about our research methods embody expectations about the nature of fieldwork and the experience of the fieldworker (chs. 7, 8). Framing participant observation as an encounter between Self and Other, between different worlds of meaning, they assume oppositions between home and field site, between the "native" social worlds of informants and observer, between the informants' knowledge and that of the anthropologist, and between conscious research and the fieldworker's own private life.

To carry out ethnographic research in my parents' field has been to confront the impossibility of keeping separate the terms of these assumed dichotomies. This work has confused the canonical distinctions between Self and Other, insider and outsider; blurred the assumed separation between research and private life; and brought out new dimensions to the use of my self as a "research instrument." My field experience resonates in unexpected, fruitful, and sometimes uncomfortable ways with my own family history. I will begin, therefore, by presenting some information about my family of origin. Then I explain how I came to do fieldwork in computer science, describing some of the resonance between family site and field site. Exploring the notion of science kinship, I next consider relations in the field as kinship relations. And finally, I consider the question of whether research in which one is positioned as science kin should be considered "real" fieldwork.

## LOCATING MYSELF AS "SCIENCE KIN"

I am the daughter, sister, granddaughter, and wife of scientists—science kin with a vengeance. My parents both studied mathematics and then went on after World War II to help develop and to teach the discipline we now know as computer science. My father, George Forsythe, was the founding chair of one of the first computer science departments in the country, located at a well-known university on the West Coast. My mother, Alexandra Forsythe, had another sort of career in science. Bright and articulate, but not given a faculty post at the university where my father flourished, she went on to introduce computer science education into the local secondary schools. She also co-authored a series of college-level textbooks on computing.

Born in 1947, I grew up in what is now Silicon Valley, dinner table witness to the construction of a discipline and a disciplinary culture. In computer science circles I was identified then—and am sometimes still—as George and Sandra's daughter. In a nuclear family composed of two computer-loving parents and one computer-loving brother, I was the odd one out—the one headed for any direction but computing. Setting out to study medicine, I discovered anthropology in college, drawn by the pleasure of interpreting problems of meaning. In graduate school, I focused on the anthropology of Europe, received a Ph.D. in 1974, and went on to spend the first decade of my professional career as a Europeanist. Most of that time, I actually lived in Europe, carrying out field studies in Scotland and Germany.

Several things about our family background contributed to what it later meant to me to undertake fieldwork in computer science. First, our household was a very intellectual place; my parents valued reason over emotion. Since they both worked a lot while at home, and often discussed their work, our home had some of the characteristics of a professional site. I received a good deal of academic training at their hands. My mother focused on teaching me writing and mathematics; I found the former more interesting. A skilled writer and editor, co-author of many textbooks on computing, she critiqued my essays and thank-you notes, urging me to write clear and straightforward prose. Also a prolific writer and editor, my father focused on careful reasoning skills.

As the youngest family member, as a female, and as someone who did not share the family bent for mathematical abstraction, I struggled to be taken seriously and to belong. Within our family, my warmest connection was with my father, whose sense of humor I shared.

As members of the Society of Friends (Quakers), my parents were committed to some distinctive values that were expressed in their work. My mother placed great importance on intellectual integrity. If she saw something as logically insupportable, she said so—whether or not it was politically advantageous to her. This reflects the Quaker injunction to "speak truth to power." She demanded a great deal of her students, her children, and herself. My father's values were also expressed in his work, articulated for example in publications and lectures urging that science not be divorced from conscience.[3] During the 1960s and early 1970s, as radical students attacked the university computer center, he did what he could to protect the machines—but also made it clear that he agreed with many of the students' concerns. An enthusiastic proponent of the computer revolution, he also urged his colleagues to be mindful of the broader social good and of the individual right to privacy.

Both of my parents died, rather young, of cancer. My mother developed breast cancer in her early forties; she died in 1980, at the age of 61. My father died in 1972, at age 55, of a rapid and incurable malignancy. Two years later, as a graduate student, my brother also developed cancer, which he survived. My parents had been liked and respected. In addition to their family, they left behind friends, colleagues, mentors, and students who missed them and remained sad about their deaths.

HOW I CAME TO DO FIELDWORK IN COMPUTER SCIENCE

In 1985, I returned to this country after ten years away and took up residence in the town where I had grown up. By then, both my parents had been dead for some years. That year, the computer science department my father

had founded celebrated its twentieth anniversary, and I was invited to the reception. There, I met an artificial intelligence (AI) researcher who had known
and liked my parents. He invited me to visit his lab. I went, was fascinated,
began to perceive some contrasts between their epistemological stance and
my own, and began an ethnographic study of this branch of computer science. For the next eight years, I was a full-time participant-observer in different settings of applied computer science. While I left full-time fieldwork
in 1994, I continue to investigate and write about the work and the epistemological world of people in various branches of computing.

## Fieldwork as a Way of Recovering My Parents

How did a casual visit to an AI lab turn into fieldwork, and why did I stay
in that site (and its successors) for the next eight years? In 1985, I was not
an anthropologist of science and technology; as far as I knew, there was no
such thing at the time. In any case, as an anthropologist, I had a different
specialty. At the time of that initial visit, I did not make a conscious decision
to study the lab or even to write a proposal for such a study. Instead, I simply came back to the lab for more visits.

In retrospect, I see that I did not begin fieldwork there as a professional
act, but rather as a personal one. At that point, I had few living relatives,
was newly separated, and had just returned to a country in which I was
something of a stranger. The departmental reception had immersed me in a
social situation that was friendly and familiar. I knew many of those present
and they knew me; at least, they knew me as George and Sandra's daughter.

Visiting the lab revealed more dimensions of familiarity. People there
seemed like my family in some ways—in their intellectual and interactional
styles, in the disciplinary world they talked about, in their fascination with
hardware and software, in their preference for technical problems rather
than social ones. Even the setting reminded me of my family home. Having
grown up surrounded by calculators and then computers, and having used
them myself since high school, I felt at home around machines. One of my
first acts upon returning to the United States had been to buy a Macintosh.

In short, the lab was emotionally resonant for me. Being around computer scientists was a way of revisiting the social and intellectual world of
my parents, a world I missed. It was also a way of encountering people who
shared my grief over their illness and death, something few people had
shared during my years in Europe. Perhaps because my childhood house-

hold had been a bit like a lab, the lab felt like home. Although I did not think of it that way at the time, turning my presence into fieldwork provided me with a way to be there.

After several visits, I engaged with the work of the lab over a procedure known as "knowledge acquisition," during which software developers gather information from "expert" informants by means of face-to-face conversation. This process was being undertaken with no training in interview technique and no discussion of the nature of knowledge or the fact that people from different disciplines may view the same thing rather differently. Not surprisingly, researchers in the lab were having trouble with knowledge acquisition; they did their best to avoid it by making the graduate students do it (ch. 3; Forsythe and Buchanan 1989). When I pointed out that anthropologists know something about interviewing and offered to share what I knew, the head of the lab suggested that I help to teach the graduate students about interview technique. After I had made informal contributions for a while, he showed me a request for proposals on knowledge acquisition and suggested that I write one. I did so, was funded, and became an official postdoc at the lab.

## Fieldwork as a Coping Mechanism

If the feeling of family familiarity made computer science in some ways a comfortable place to be, it also evoked some uncomfortable feelings grounded in my family of origin. Chief among these was the struggle to belong, to be accepted as an insider among scientists. As an anthropologist in the lab, I was clearly marginal. Some people openly wondered what I was doing there and why the head of the lab encouraged my presence. I sometimes felt patronized by people who could not understand what a "soft" social scientist was doing among "hard scientists" like them. Qualitative researchers get little respect in computer science and engineering, fields in which "technical knowledge" is not understood to refer to what anthropologists know.[4] Twelve years later, my name is on nine publications in computer science, engineering, and medical informatics, but I am still regarded in these fields as having no technical qualifications.

In the male world of computer science, I sometimes felt invisible because of my gender as well as my discipline. The department where I started out had no female faculty members and had never tenured a full-time woman. In the group of soft-money labs to which "my" lab belonged was only one other woman past the doctorate—a spectacularly intelligent and productive researcher who hit the glass ceiling when she sought a hard-money position. Early on, she commented to me that I had no long-term prospects in the lab. As she put it, they would keep me around for a while "like an exotic butterfly" but would never take me seriously.

Being around computer science, then, was rewarding in some ways and painful in others. On the one hand, it evoked familiar memories of our "family business" and provided a site for the shared expression of emotion concerning my parents. It was also highly stimulating from an intellectual standpoint. Bright and opinionated, computer scientists are fun to study. On the other hand, the feeling of marginality as a female anthropologist in this setting was difficult to tolerate in the long run.

These multiple valences were not fully evident in the beginning; it took me years to sort out the story I am telling. At the same time, something—presumably the emotional resonance of the setting itself—led me to launch more or less automatically into familiar routines of elicitation, comparison, and analysis. The secure identity of ethnographic observer and its associated epistemological disciplines acted as a coping mechanism, helping to create some emotional distance and intellectual order in a situation that was both seductive and confusing. This allowed me to handle the feeling of marginality by professionalizing it, framing the situation as the legitimately distanced relationship between anthropologist and informants.

Every participant-observer feels marginal, at least some of the time. The ability to tolerate and profit from that position is a prerequisite for doing ethnography. During years of fieldwork in Scotland and Germany, I was able to live with that feeling. Despite the normal yearning to belong to my informants' communities, I knew I was an outsider. In the lab, in contrast, I felt on some level that I really *should* belong; because of the resonance between my family of origin and the world of the lab, marginality felt much more painful. In addition, I stayed in the lab and its successors for a very long time, entrapped perhaps by this struggle. When in 1994 I finally decided to return to a base in anthropology, the relief was considerable.

GEORGE'S DAUGHTER, ROBERT'S GIRL: FIELDWORK
    AS KIN RELATIONSHIP

Since the notion of science kin plays on anthropological representations of relatedness within the family structure, I turn now to the question of kinship. Within my family of origin, I related to other family members as child, sister, and daughter. At the time I began work in computer science, I was 37, thirteen years past the doctorate, and a seasoned fieldworker. However, the nature of participant observation as a research method in combination with particular characteristics of this field situation helped to frame me within the lab in the role of daughter.

Participant observation depends on the metaphor of socialization: constructing herself as a notional child, the fieldworker asks the informants to teach her to behave and interpret things as they would. This method exploits what Germans call *Narrenfreiheit*—the freedom accorded to fools and children to make mistakes and ask questions about almost anything. In setting out to learn about the work of the lab through this technique, I positioned myself as fictive child in relation to the expertise that defined the disciplinary setting. This aspect of the situation was reinforced for me, at least, by the location of the field site. My first two years of fieldwork took place in a part of the department my father had founded, on a campus I had known as a teenager. There, the name Forsythe defined me as George and Sandra's daughter. Thus, in a setting full of cues from my youth, and by virtue of my relationship as a daughter, I gained entrée to (what became) the field.

## Robert's Daughter

I first visited the lab at the invitation of the lab head and remained there under his protection. This man, whom I will call Robert, became a mentor and friend, and remained so throughout my eight years in his world. Without his interest and support, there would have been no fieldwork.

Although Robert is only a few years older than I, our relationship had something of a father-daughter tone. Part of that is his personal style, as a kind individual who relates to many people in a benign and fatherly sort of way. He reminded me of my father, both in his gentle, thoughtful manner and in the fact that he seemed to enjoy my questions and insights about his field. Anomalous himself in having been trained as a philosopher rather than as a computer scientist, mathematician, or engineer, Robert was sympathetic to my interest in seeking out underlying assumptions and in taking a broad view of issues that his colleagues often looked at more narrowly.

In addition, as an AI researcher, Robert explicitly enjoys intelligence; he labels certain people as "very smart," and was kind enough to include me in that category. Again, this evoked memories of my parents, who had related to me largely as a developing intellect and had valued me for my intelligence. Just as I found it intellectually interesting to study Robert and his fellow researchers, I think he found it interesting to analyze my ideas and assumptions. Over time, as I learned to predict what he and other informants would say in certain situations, he in turn formulated a predictive model of what I would say.

Like all the labs I investigated, Robert's was structured hierarchically. He was senior in his field, whereas I was a rank beginner. Over time, as I realized that anthropology could usefully be applied in AI, I began to function as more of a colleague. Nevertheless, in the lab structure, I was always junior to him, always identified as one of "his" researchers. That possessive description is characteristic of the field. Different research groups are known for taking different approaches to creating machine intelligence; these differences can be quite ideological, are passed down to students and junior colleagues, and are viewed as defining separate communities within the field. To come from Robert's lab was to be understood as belonging to a particular section of the AI community: not someone, for example, who did robotics or neural nets. Thus, my informants themselves understood lab membership in kinship-like terms, as implying a certain kind of inheritance—an assumed shaping by the parental figure of the lab head.

Finally, my sense of being a daughter in the lab was reinforced by gender issues.

## *Sandra's Daughter*

As others have noted (Female Graduate Students 1983; Pearl, Pollack, Riskin, Thomas, Wolf, and Wu 1990), and as I have described elsewhere (ch. 11), computer science and its constituent fields (e.g., AI and medical informatics) are not without sexism. In the computer science arenas I studied, it is normal to define female researchers in relation to men—typically those who trained them or in whose research group they work.[5]

This gender-based treatment provided another source of resonance between the lab and my family of origin. My mother's long struggle to be taken seriously as a computer scientist was replayed for me in my own marginality. This became clear to me when I set out to write a paper about the deletion of women in computer science. Struggling to turn my own field experience into text, I found myself writing again and again about my mother. Thus, research in the lab also showed me to myself as Sandra's daughter.

I have argued that women in computer science labs are framed in a sense as kin dependents of the senior male lab head. My self-presentation as a junior "learner" and the fact that Robert reminded me of my own father helped me to fit into this aspect of disciplinary culture. Over time, however, this role as fictive daughter became uncomfortable. Being taken less than seriously as a woman and as a "non-technical" social scientist was irritating to my sense of competence as a professional anthropologist. I wanted increasingly to be treated as a grown-up.

## SCIENCE KINSHIP AND THE ANTHROPOLOGICAL FIELDWORK CANON

When I first began writing about my fieldwork in computer science, I described it simply as fieldwork. Having used ethnographic methods to study Scots and Germans, I saw myself as using these same methods to study scientists. To some extent, this was true: ethnography among scientists has many things in common with ethnography in other settings. Certainly my own previous field experience was enormously helpful as I invented my own approach to studying the work and epistemology of software development.

From another standpoint, however, this was not a conventional anthropological study. While I did not consciously set out to create this state of affairs and was not fully aware of it for a long time, this fieldwork was personal to me in a way that my previous research was not. In many ways, this was rewarding. On the other hand, it was sometimes quite harrowing for me personally. My continuing project of going through the twenty-four cartons of my parents' collected papers in the university archives has been surprisingly painful. Most of this material is from my father, who documented his every professional act. Letters and memos in his files confront me again and again with reminders of the plans and dreams curtailed by his sudden death.

## Collapsing Assumed Dichotomies

The idealized dichotomies that characterize our fieldwork canon have been challenged by feminists and by anthropologists of technoscience (chs. 7, 8; Behar 1993; Behar and Gordon 1995; Paget 1988, 1993; Traweek 1988a, 1992). To study technoscience in one's own society is inevitably to encounter informants very like ourselves—possibly university faculty members, certainly literate, and probably powerful. Such informants may be our own colleagues, employers, or competitors (ch. 8), whose work may intersect quite strongly with our own lives. Perhaps the most memorable account of such intersection appears in the work of the late medical sociologist Marianne (Tracy) Paget. Having published a fine ethnographic study on the inevitability of mistakes in medical practice (Paget 1988), Paget addressed the same territory again five years later from her changed position as the victim of a serious medical error (Paget 1993).

The probability that a strict distinction can be maintained between Self and Other, field site and home, is even further eroded for science kin, whose informants may resemble their own relatives. In my own case, fieldwork in technoscience brought me literally face to face with some of my parents' friends and colleagues—a state of affairs in which at least some of the dichotomies assumed in the fieldwork canon broke down completely.

DISCUSSION

How should my years of research in computer science be characterized? Was this a personal journey or was it anthropological field research? Who was I in relation to my informants—insider or outsider, "techie" or anthropologist, subject or object? And who were my informants in relation to me? What about our epistemological categories—what does "scientific knowledge" mean if it includes things I learned as a child at the dinner table? Clearly, the experience of science kin who do fieldwork in technoscience destabilizes the internal logic of the fieldwork canon. If to do fieldwork is to travel *away* from home, outside of our native worlds of experience, into novel systems of knowledge and meaning, then by implication, real research cannot be personal.

Nevertheless, I would argue that what I did was both personal journey and genuine field research. During those eight years, I did indeed revisit various struggles from my family of origin. At the same time, I carried out innovative and productive ethnographic research. I wrote and contributed to funded proposals amounting to several million dollars, and I learned and wrote a good deal about epistemology and practice in AI and medical informatics. In so doing, I helped to create the field we now know as the anthropology of science and technology and to broaden the anthropology of work to include the work of doing science.

While I have mentioned the personal frustration of not being considered a "real" computer scientist, I should point out that in this research, I actually achieved a much greater degree of participation in the informant community than is usual in ethnographic work. Like some other anthropologists of technoscience (e.g., Traweek, Suchman, Heath), I have some professional standing in the scientific communities I studied. In medical informatics (a field at the intersection of computer science and medicine), I am regularly invited to review journal manuscripts as well as to chair sessions and present talks at AMIA (the American Medical Informatics Association). I continue to publish in the field, do some consulting, and have been asked to write tenure letters for candidates in both medical informatics and AI.

To acknowledge that this work was both personal and professional is to dissolve the normative boundary between personal life and intentional fieldwork. But is this really so anomalous? All anthropologists bring to their work experiences and attitudes learned in childhood; we often make choices about what and where to study that have personal meaning for us. For example, my decisions to do fieldwork in Scotland and Germany reflected in part an interest in my own Scottish and German heritage. The idealized fieldwork narrative fails to acknowledge that the personal and professional overlap in ethnographic work of many kinds. Since technoscience is closer to home in several senses than some more conventional field sites, the potential for overlap between personal life and field site may be greater for anthropologists of science and technology. For science kin, especially, that overlap can be dramatic. In my view, however, this difference is a matter of degree rather than kind.

## Is Being Science Kin an Advantage or a Disadvantage?

Finally, I want to raise the question of whether being science kin is an advantage or a disadvantage for doing fieldwork in a scientific setting. In my experience, it was both. With respect to both logistics and the experiential problem of "seeing," my fieldwork was at the same time helped and hindered by my position as science kin.

It certainly helped with access to the field; I was invited to the lab in the first place because of a personal connection, and I imagine that this connection helped to sustain the relationship in the time before I began to produce grant money and publications. On the other hand, being science kin was also a constraint. For example, it limited my freedom to define myself; in my initial lab, at least, certain things seemed to be assumed or expected of me because I was George and Sandra's daughter. For example, on one occasion, I tried to donate copies of my parents' books to a departmental computer science library. But the lab administrator looked at me with such horror that I took the books away again, although I had multiple copies of each at home. Clearly, I was expected to keep my parents' books.

My status as a sort of computer science princess may also have amplified a few reactions when I began publishing critique. While anthropologists of science and technology tend to see critique as part of our work, computer scientists are used to being taken very seriously. Although I have been discreet and although I invite Robert's comments on everything I write, not everyone in computer science has been pleased with my analyses of their practice. One or two people who knew my parents have over time become rather hostile. I sometimes wonder if they see my work as a betrayal of my family heritage. In contrast, I see my critique as consistent with my parents' concern with intellectual integrity and with the social and political implications of computer usage. In urging people to consider whether what they are building into intelligent systems is truly in the interest of users, I believe that I am carrying on their legacy, using my anthropology to "speak truth to power."

With respect to epistemological issues, I also found my position as science kin to be both advantageous and disadvantageous. In what we have been taught to see as "normal" fieldwork, the anthropologist faces the task of making the strange familiar. In contrast, anthropologists of technoscience often have the opposite problem. When dealing with informants very like oneself, a major challenge is to make the familiar strange enough to be able to "see" it. This can be a problem for science kin.

In some ways, my computer science informants resembled my family; I recognized certain assumptions and reasoning styles from conversations with my parents and older brother. In one sense, then, this background helped me to understand my informants' worldview, although I did not always share it. At the same, that overlap could be confusing: I was not always sure whether I knew something from observing system designers or from having picked it up at the dinner table.[6] While this overlap between childhood knowledge and knowledge gained in the field blurs boundaries assumed in the canon, it is also a source of enrichment. The background I brought into the field increased my understanding of what I learned in the lab and helped me to know my informants as people.

In sum, while anthropology's normative fieldwork narrative implies that the ethnographic stance requires strict separation between personal life and formal research, the work of science kin demonstrates that it is possible to do useful fieldwork when personal life and research sphere intertwine. In fact, I would argue that in science and technology studies, science kin have a certain advantage over other fieldworkers in that they may find it easier to maintain some degree of critical distance from the views of their informants. Perhaps because science is the source of some of our society's most sacred truths, I observe a tendency on the part of some researchers in science and technology studies to accept their informants' assertions without question. In contrast, those of us who have known scientists all our lives as relatives and fallible human beings may be less likely to accept their every word as gospel and, thus, more able to maintain the ethnographic stance upon which fieldwork depends.

The following list includes publications by Diana Forsythe that are not included in this book and not referenced in the bibliography.

## Studies of Knowledge-Based Systems and Medical Informatics

Aydin, C. E., and D. E. Forsythe
1997 "Implementing Computers in Ambulatory Care: Implications of Practice Patterns for System Design." *Proceedings of the American Medical Informatics Association Annual Fall Symposium* 21: 677–81.
Bhavnani, S., U. Flemming, D. E. Forsythe, J. Garrett, D. S. Shaw, and A. Tsai
1995 "Understanding and Assisting CAD Users in the Real World." In L. N. Kalisperis and B. Kolarevic (eds.), *Computing in Design: Enabling, Capturing, and Sharing Ideas*. Proceedings of Association for Computer Aided Design in Architecture. State College, Penn.: Nittany Valley Offset. Pp. 209–27.
1996 "CAD Usage in an Architectural Office: From Observations to Active Assistance." *Automation in Construction* 5: 243–55.
Buchanan, B. G., J. D. Moore, D. E. Forsythe, G. Banks, and S. Ohlsson
1992 "Involving Patients in Health Care: Using Medical Informatics for Explanation in the Clinical Setting." In M. E. Frisse (ed.), *Proceedings of the Sixteenth Symposium on Computer Applications in Medical Care*. New York: McGraw-Hill. Pp. 510–4.
Forsythe, D. E.
1992 "Using Ethnography to Build a Working System: Rethinking Basic Design Assumptions." In M. E. Frisse (ed.), *Proceedings of the Sixteenth Symposium on Computer Applications in Medical Care*. New York: McGraw-Hill. Pp. 505–9.
1993 Review of *Women, Information Technology, and Scholarship*, by H. J. Taylor, C. Kramarae, and M. Ebben (eds.). *Science, Technology, and Human Values* 20 (1): 108–10.
1998 "Using Ethnography to Investigate Life Scientists' Information Needs." *Bulletin of the Medical Library Association* 86: 402–9.

1998 "An Anthropologist's Viewpoint: Observations and Commentary Regarding 'Implementation of Nursing Vocabularies in Computer-based Systems.'" *Journal of the American Medical Informatics Association* 4: 329–31.

## European Studies

Forsythe, D. E.

1974 *Escape to Fulfillment: Urban-Rural Migration and the Future of a Small Island Community*. Ph.D. diss., Anthropology Department, Cornell University.

1980 "Urban Incomers and Rural Change: The Impact of Migrants from the City on Life in an Orkney Community." *Sociologia Ruralis* 20 (4): 287–307.

1981 "The Social Value of Rural Schools: National Ideology, Local Perceptions, and Regional Decision-Making." In A. Jackson (ed.), *Way of Life: Dominant Ideologies and Local Communities*. London: Social Science Research Council, North Sea Oil Panel Occasional Paper No. 11. Pp. 32–47.

1981 "Urban-Rural Migration and the Pastoral Ideal: An Orkney Case." In A. Jackson (ed.), *Integration and Immigration*. London: Social Science Research Council, North Sea Oil Panel Occasional Paper No. 12. Pp. 22–45.

1982 "Gross Migration and Social Change: An Orkney Case." In H. Jones (ed.), *Recent Migration in Northern Scotland: Pattern, Process, and Impact*. London: Social Science Research Council, North Sea Oil Panel Occasional Paper No. 13. Pp. 90–103.

1982 *Urban-Rural Migration: Change and Conflict in an Orkney Island Community*. London: Social Science Research Council, North Sea Oil Panel Occasional Paper, No. 14.

1983 "Planning Implications of Urban-Rural Migration." *Gloucestershire Papers in Local and Regional Planning*, No. 21, October.

1983 "Review." *Sociologia Ruralis* 23 (3/4): 299–301.

1983 "Urban-Rural Migration and Local Development: An Orkney Case." In J. C. Hansen, J. Naustdalslid, and J. Sewel (eds.), *Centre-Periphery: Theory and Practice*. Sogndal, Norway: Sogn- and Fjordane Regional College. Pp. 232–45.

1984 "Deutschland als wenig erforschtes Gebiet: Ein Problem in der Ethnologie Westeuropas." (Germany as an Under-Studied Area: A Problem of the Anthropology of Western Europe.) *Kölner Zeitschrift für Soziologie und Sozialpsychologie* 26: 124–40.

1984 "The Social Effects of Primary School Closure." In P. Lowe and T. Bradley (eds.), *Rurality and Locality: Economy and Society in Rural Regions*. Norwich, U.K.: Geo-Books. Pp. 209–24.

1984 "The Social Impact of the New Urban-Rural Migration on One of the Orkney Islands." *Northern Scotland* 6 (1): 63–70.

Forsythe, D. E., with I. Carter, G. A. MacKay, J. Nisbet, P. Sadler, J. Sewel, D. Shanks, and J. Welsh

1983 *The Rural Community and the Small School*. Aberdeen, Scotland: Aberdeen University Press.

REFERENCE MATTER

## 1. Blaming the User in Medical Informatics

1. Earlier versions of this paper were presented to the Society for Social Studies of Science, Cambridge, Mass., November 16, 1991, and to the American Anthropological Association, Chicago, Ill., November 23, 1991. Some of the material in this paper appeared in Forsythe and Buchanan (1991). I wish to thank my anonymous informants for their help and patience. For editorial suggestions, I also thank P. Agre, D. Hess, and J. Nyce.

2. The insight that scientific practice can usefully be viewed as work derives from Star (1989).

3. The ACMI meeting was held February 3–5, 1991, in Palm Springs, California. The theme of the meeting was "Modularization, Sharing, and Integration: A Medical Informatics Agenda for the Decade." When I asked an informant to explain the relationship between ACMI and AMIA (the American Medical Informatics Association), the main professional association in medical informatics, he replied (of ACMI), "It's the old boys!"

4. Sometimes this is supplemented by information derived from uncontrolled "experiments" in which experts are asked to perform contrived tasks outside their normal work settings. This simulated work is generally taken as representative of real-world work, an assumption that I have questioned elsewhere (see ch. 2).

5. For a broader discussion of the hard/soft split in relation to AI, see Edwards (1990).

6. I am indebted to Traweek's analysis of the embedding of scientists' values in the tools they construct (1988a).

7. Marginal figures do exist on the fringes of medical informatics. Although their unorthodox systems are apparently no less appealing to users than those of their more orthodox colleagues, they hold little power and receive little institutional support.

8. A similar comment is made by Bader and Nyce (1991).

## 2. The Construction of Work in Artificial Intelligence

1. I thank B. G. Buchanan, D. Hess, B. Kuipers, L. Layne, F. Provost, B. Shen, J. Singleton, S. L. Star, my anonymous informants, and the anonymous reviewers for their helpful comments on earlier drafts of this paper. I also thank S. Cozzens for being such a patient and supportive editor. A previous version of the paper was presented to the Society for Social Studies of Science, Minneapolis, on October 20, 1990. This research is supported by National Library of Medicine grant LM05299-02.

2. Rule-based expert systems and knowledge engineering do not constitute the entire field of AI. However, since my participant observation has taken place mainly within that world, my generalizations should be understood in that context. One major alternative approach to system-building within AI (as opposed to such other research areas as robotics) is defined by the system architecture known variously as *connectionism, neural nets*, or *PDP* (parallel and distributed processing). Adherents of these two approaches compete for funding and for the power to define what should count as "real AI."

3. Expert systems are a subset of the broader category of knowledge-based systems. Further information on expert systems is provided in the following sources: Davis (1989); Harmon and King (1985); Hayes-Roth, Waterman, and Lenat (1983); Johnson (1986); Scott, Clayton, and Gibson (1991); Waterman (1986).

4. This metaphor is generally attributed to E. A. Feigenbaum.

5. See Gasser (1986) for discussion of this and others ways in which users "manage" computer systems in order to work around design problems.

6. The study of the meaning of "information" was conducted with special reference to the way this term is constructed in medical informatics, a field that lies at the intersection of computer science, information science, and medicine.

7. On other occasions in the course of my fieldwork I have encountered further examples of the use of particular technical skills as boundary markers. In three of the laboratories in which I have done research, I was assigned a computer terminal or networked personal computer at which to work. In each case, knowledge of the local operating system (different in each laboratory) seemed to convey a message about belonging in some way to the lab. Informants became discernibly more friendly and helpful once I had demonstrated the ability to use the local e-mail and text editing software with some degree of facility. The text editors of relevance here are those which (like Emacs and vi) are necessary for "system hacking," that is, working on large computer operating systems. Knowledge of such user-friendly personal word processors as Word or MacWrite does not carry the same symbolic meaning.

8. For further anthropological analysis of the knowledge elicitation process, see ch. 3 and Forsythe and Buchanan (1989). For discussion of knowledge elicitation from a different point of view, see Collins (1990). My reactions to Collins's discussion of knowledge engineering are given in chapter 3.

9. A similar observation is reported in a case study by Blomberg and Henderson (1990). They note that even in a participatory design project explicitly intended to

involve users in the design of a computer-based system, designers of the computer interface ended up relying "not on seeing use, but on talking about it" (1990: 357).

10. I have observed this to be the case in the course of my own ongoing fieldwork in Pittsburgh in settings in internal medicine, neurology, and emergency medicine.

## 3. Engineering Knowledge

1. I wish to express my gratitude and respect to the knowledge engineers at the lab as well as other members of the AI community for their patience and their help. Knowing that I do not always agree with them, they have continued to support my work. Outside of AI, I thank D. Edge, P. Edwards, J. Fujimura, L. Gasser, D. Hess, D. Joravsky, L. Layne, M. Lynch, T. Pinch, B. Shen, J. Singleton, P. Slezak, S. L. Star, A. Strauss, L. Suchman, P. Taylor, D. Turnbull, S. Zabusky, and the anonymous reviewers for helpful comments and suggestions. Earlier versions of this paper were presented at the twelfth annual meeting of the Society for Social Studies of Science, Worcester, Massachusetts, in 1987; at the Department of Science and Technology Studies, Rensselaer Polytechnic Institute, in 1990; and at the Program in Science, Technology and Society, Cornell University, in 1991. This research is supported by National Library of Medicine grant LM05299-02.

2. See, for example, Collins (1987a, 1990), Dreyfus (1979), Dreyfus and Dreyfus (1986), Weizenbaum (1976), and Winograd and Flores (1986).

3. Further information on expert systems is provided in Harmon and King (1985), Hayes-Roth, Waterman, and Lenat (1983), Johnson (1986), and Scott, Clayton, and Gibson (1991).

4. For an ethnographic example of this, see Geertz (1973: ch. 6).

5. This parallel has also been noted by others within the social science community. See Collins (1987b), Werner (1988), and Benfer and Furbee (1989).

6. For example, see Cassell and Jacobs (1987), Geertz (1988), and Marcus and Fischer (1986).

7. Rule-based expert systems and knowledge engineering do not constitute the entire field of AI. However, since my participant observation has taken place mainly within that world, my generalizations should be understood in that context. The major alternative approach to system-building within AI (as opposed to such other research areas as robotics) is defined by the system architecture known variously as *connectionism*, *neural nets*, or *PDP* (parallel and distributed processing). Adherents of these two approaches compete for funding and for the power to define what should count as "real AI" (see ch. 6).

8. Forsythe has a footnote indicating that the first four paragraphs that appear in this section are drawn from the first paragraphs of the introduction to what is now chapter 1. Because the essay is included in this volume, the redundant paragraphs are omitted—ed.

9. (The journal is significant because the Fleck-Forsythe debate that appears here is in the same journal—ed.) See the Symposium on "Computer Discovery and the

Sociology of Scientific Knowledge" (*Social Studies of Science*, vol. 19, no. 4, November 1989, pp. 563–694), containing contributions by H. M Collins, S. Fuller, R. Giere, M. Gorman, G. Myers, P. Slezak, P. Thagard, S. Woolgar, and G. Myers; and "Responses and Replies" to this Symposium (*Social Studies of Science*, vol. 21, no. 1, February 1991, pp. 143–56), containing contributions by H. M Collins, S. Fuller, R. Giere, M. Gorman, H. Simon, and P. Slezak. The debate continued face-to-face in the course of contributions by H. M Collins, H. Dreyfus, S. Fuller, M. Gorman, and P. Slezak during sessions presented to the Society for Social Studies of Science, Boston, Massachusetts, November 14–7, 1991. See also the debate between H. Dreyfus and H. Collins in *Social Studies of Science* (vol. 22, no. 4, 1994, 717–39) and between P. Slezak (1992) and H. Collins (1992).

10. In his 1990 book, Collins uses the word "culture" but does not define the concept. In contrast to the anthropological usage adopted in this paper, he seems to view culture as an invariant part of the general surround, like air. Thus, he treats "cultural skills" as simply present or absent rather than considering *which* cultural tradition defines what will be taken as skill in a particular context (e.g., Collins 1990: 109). In general, Collins overlooks cultural issues, often supporting his generalizations with convenient fictional examples (e.g., "data" from "laser society" with its "culture of lasers and electricity," p. 113) rather than examples from the real world. When he does offer real-world examples, they tend to involve his own experience, from which he generalizes broadly. The resultant acultural perspective is illustrated by the assertion that "Nowadays, everyone knows how to put money in a pinball machine and how to make the balls run" (p. 107). Such statements ignore the differences in knowledge and experience (contingent upon gender, social class, ethnicity, etc.) that contribute to cultural variation within Collins' own society, let alone the vast cultural diversity within the universal framework of human experience implied by the word "everyone." What one suspects the statement to mean is that *Collins* knows how to operate a pinball machine. This approach resembles the "I am the world" reasoning characteristic of the knowledge engineers described in this paper (see section on reification of knowledge).

11. Collins' detailed account (1990: 135–78) of his own attempt to build an expert system sheds little light on the everyday work practices of professional knowledge engineers. Note that Slezak (1992) and Collins (1992) each cite my work in disputing each other's arguments.

12. These and many other expert systems are described in the extensive catalog of expert systems included in Waterman, who also provides citations to the AI literature for each system. See Waterman (1986: 244–99).

13. For example, see Collins, Green, and Draper (1985); Collins (1987a, 1987b, 1990); and Suchman (1987). Not every social scientist has reacted in this way, however. For example, Werner has long been enthusiastic about the idea of developing expert systems to facilitate research in ethnoscience (a branch of linguistic anthropology), noting that "cultural knowledge is so vast that work in this area is unrealistic without machine aid" (Werner 1972: 272). See also Werner (1978, 1988).

14. Although Suchman and Collins address the problem of knowledge, they have

not analyzed the knowledge acquisition problem per se. Collins' account (1990: 135–78) of his own problems with knowledge elicitation is not an analysis of the problem. Thus, I am inferring a bit from their writing.

15. Personal communication, E. Gerson, September 6, 1987.

16. Both Collins (1987a) and Buchanan and I (Forsythe and Buchanan 1989) have suggested that knowledge elicitation would benefit if knowledge engineers made use of participant observation as well as interviews.

17. Quotations for which no citation is provided are verbatim quotations from informants in the Lab.

18. From the text of an advertisement for a video course entitled "Expert Systems: Automating Knowledge Acquisition," distributed by Addison-Wesley at the annual meeting of the American Association for Artificial Intelligence, Seattle, Washington, July 1987.

19. Kidd (1987: 2–3) comments critically on the "mining analogy" used by Feigenbaum and McCorduck (1984).

20. By "methodology" I refer here not to the use of specific interviewing techniques (e.g., the repertory grid technique described by Shaw and Gaines [1987]), but rather to the recognition that interviewing requires a systematic approach to factors—such as planning, organization, question formulation, cross-checking, data-recording, and post-interview evaluation—that are not part of everyday conversation. This information is contained in any good introductory textbook on interviewing and may well be common sense to a social scientist. However, the knowledge engineers' commonsense approach does not include systematic attention to such factors. For the repertory grid technique, see Shaw and Gaines (1987). For introductory material on interviewing, see R. Gordon (1987), Kahn and Cannell (1961), or Werner and Schoepfle (1987).

21. For an attempt to convey this point with reference to some issues in medical informatics, a major application area of AI, see Forsythe, Buchanan, Osheroff, and Miller (1992).

22. Personal communication. I have heard Leigh Star make this point in many discussions. (See also Star 1991—ed.)

23. Turkle (1988: 252; 1989) has argued that AI based upon neural net architecture (to which she refers as "emergent AI") is not subject to the limitations of AI based upon the rule-based systems approach (to which she refers as the "information-processing model"). I differ with Turkle on this point: in my view the selectivity of the knowledge represented in a system remains problematic, no matter which architecture is used to represent that knowledge. See Forsythe (1989a).

24. The class, gender, ethnic, and political biases of AI and the computing world in general have been addressed from both within and without. See Perry and Greber (1990); Turkle and Papert (1990); Kramer and Lehmen (1990); Pearl, Pollack, Riskin, Thomas, Wolf, and Wu (1990); Female Graduate Students (1983); and Edwards (1990).

25. This term [muted voices] is borrowed from Shirley Ardener's discussion (1975: vii–xxiii) of the muting of women's voices.

## 4. Knowing Engineers?

1. The arguments usually take the form of a dichotomy: for example, "arithmo-morphic"/"dialectical," as in Georgescu-Roegen (1971); "algorithmic"/"encultura-tional," as in Collins (1987b); and "mentalism"/"strong program" in the sociology of knowledge, as exemplified in many passages of the symposium on "Computer Discovery and the Sociology of Knowledge" (Social Studies of Science, vol. 21, no. 1 [February 1991], pp. 143–56) and further comments in Social Studies of Science (vol. 21, no. 1 [February 1991], pp. 143–56).

2. Steve Woolgar has made similar observations: "Despite the vigor of the socio-logical challenge, I suggest that the sociologists' commitment to particular modes of representation ultimately imposes severe limitations on the likely success of their at-tack on cognitivism" (Woolgar 1987: 312).

3. This is a paraphrase of a common complaint. For more extended examples of partisan expression from AI proponents, although not expressed in inclusive/exclu-sive pronoun terms, see the symposium cited in note 1.

4. This term ("actants") has become widely used through the work of Latour and his colleagues. See, for example, Callon, Law, and Rip (1986); Latour (1987); Latour, Mauguin, and Teil (1992).

5. This is not to deny that a critical analysis would not be worthwhile in itself. But it is a matter for analysis with reference to practical examples, within a framework providing explicit criteria, rather than slipped in as an anthropological investigation.

6. Though admittedly some do, especially those self-appointed proponents of grand programmatic claims: an example, perhaps, is Slezak (1989). In other cases, as Law (1987) has pointed out, successful engineers are precisely those able to organize and manipulate the social for their own ends, and consequently are not "deleting the social."

7. Or, as Collins (1987b) has suggested, to use AI as an "experimental probe."

8. Such as symmetry with respect to explaining truth and falsity, as argued by Bloor (1976) or symmetry between the animate and inanimate, as suggested by Cal-lon (1987).

9. Symposium on "Computer Discovery and the Sociology of Scientific Knowl-edge" (Social Studies of Science, vol. 19, no. 4 [November 1989], pp. 563–694).

10. And I advisedly mean "we" in the completely inclusive sense here. I am not at present aware of any sufficiently intelligent non-human agents!

## 5. STS (Re)constructs Anthropology

1. I am grateful to B. G. Buchanan, D. Hess, B. Shen, and S. L. Star for their comments and suggestions on earlier drafts of this paper. The acronym STS in the ti-tle refers to science and technology studies.

2. This comment is from Fleck's written review of my paper for Social Studies of Science in 1988 and 1992. In 1988, when an earlier version of "Engineering Knowl-

edge" was unsuccessfully submitted to this journal, James Fleck was the most critical of its three referees. This was my first contact with his work. When, in 1992, after further fieldwork, I submitted a revised and expanded version of the paper, Fleck
was again the most critical of the referees. However, the overall verdict was now positive—although Fleck's comments on the revised paper were identical to his comments on the original. The editors considered that his position was worth publishing
for a wider audience, in the hope of initiating a fruitful discussion, and so encouraged him to base a response on his referee's report.

3. People trained in other disciplines sometimes borrow anthropological data-
gathering methods (or aspects of these methods) without also borrowing the associated conceptual stance. Anthropologists tend to see this as problematic because we
view ethnography as a way of seeing as well as a way of gathering data. I am indebted
to D. Hess for applying the term "appropriation" to this situation (personal communication, May 17, 1993.) For examples of what might be considered appropriation,
see Latour and Woolgar (1986) and Abir-Am (1992). For an anthropologist's reaction
to the latter, see Gusterson (1992). (The examples are Forsythe's, not mine—ed.)

## 6. Artificial Intelligence Invents Itself

1. I am grateful to the knowledge engineers for their patience and help. In the social science community, I thank Elihu Gerson and Gerhard Schutte for helpful discussions of material presented here. An earlier version of this paper was presented to
the thirteenth annual meeting of the Society for Social Studies of Science, Amsterdam, in November 1988. The research reported here was funded by U.S. West.

2. Like many disciplines, AI has various camps and perspectives that are to some
extent allied with particular institutional bases. Although I refer here on occasion to
AI as a discipline, the reader should understand that unless otherwise noted, I am
writing about AI as seen by knowledge engineers in the particular laboratories that
I have studied. To protect the privacy of my informants, I refrain from naming those
labs and am purposely vague about certain details concerning them.

3. The unattributed quotations included in the text are verbatim quotations from
my informants, collected during field research.

4. For an example of other anthropological work utilizing this concept of identity, see Forsythe (1989b).

5. Source: call for nominations for the "IJCAI award for research excellence,"
circulated on the Arpanet on June 21, 1988. IJCAI (International Joint Conference
on Artificial Intelligence) is an important professional body.

6. Source: contribution from Marvin Minsky to AIList Digest, a computer bulletin board distributed on Arpanet, on July 30, 1987.

7. Source: contribution from Michael Wilson to AIList Digest, a computer bulletin board distributed on the Arpanet, on August 28, 1987.

8. Building an expert system typically involves carrying out the following steps:
(1) collecting information from one or more human informants and/or from docu-

mentary sources; (2) ordering information into procedures (e.g., rules and constraints) relevant to the operations that the prospective system is intended to perform; and (3) designing or adapting a computer program to apply these rules and constraints in performing the designated operations. The first two steps in this series—that is, the gathering of information and its translation into machine-readable form—comprise the process known as "knowledge acquisition." Knowledge engineers are regarded as specialists in this task. The early stages of knowledge acquisition often include extended face-to-face interviewing of one or more experts by the knowledge engineer(s). I refer to this interview process as "knowledge elicitation." The entire process of building expert systems appears to social scientists to be an exercise in multiple translation (see ch. 3).

9. For further information on this approach to building expert systems, see Hayes-Roth, Waterman, and Lenat (1983).

10. For further information on this approach to building expert systems, see Howard and Matheson (1984).

## 7. New Bottles, Old Wine

1. This project was funded by National Library of Medicine grant LM05299-R01 (B. G. Buchanan, PI). Contents of the paper are solely the responsibility of the author and do not represent the official views of the National Library of Medicine or of other members of the project team. I thank the latter for allowing me to carry out the work reported here. Earlier versions of this paper were presented to the workshop on Vital Signs: Cultural Perspectives on Coding Life and Vitalizing Code, organized by Joan Fujimura, at Stanford University, June 2–4, 1994; and to the Society for Social Studies of Science, New Orleans, October 12–16, 1994. For helpful comments, I am grateful to Gay Becker, Marc Berg, Patti Brennan, Bruce Buchanan, Monica Casper, Donna Haraway, Bonnie Kaplan, Susan Kelly, Barbara Koenig, Jim Nyce, Tom Rosenal, Bern Shen, Leigh Star, the conference participants, the anonymous reviewers, and the editorial staff of *Medical Anthropology Quarterly*.

2. The development of MYCIN, the first intelligent system for medicine, is described in Buchanan and Shortliffe (1984).

3. The title of this article reverses the New Testament warning against putting new wine in old bottles (Mark 1:22). It is meant to draw attention to the distinction between the character of particular technologies (which may be highly innovative) and the nature of the knowledge represented in them (which—as I show in this paper—may not be innovative at all).

4. In some institutions, this field is known as medical information science. For an overview of medical informatics as seen by its practitioners, see Shortliffe, Perreault, Wiederhold, and Fagan (1990).

5. In computer science "natural language" denotes normal, everyday language as opposed to specialized programming language. The migraine system is designed to generate explanations comprehensible to any adult English speaker.

6. Myra Brostoff and Linda Purinton (graduate students in anthropology) and Nancy Bee (research assistant in psychology) took part in and made important contributions to our ethnographic study of migraine sufferers and neurologists.

7. Taken from an unpublished project paper, this is one version of the narrative produced by research team members to explain what the migraine system was for.

8. The hyphenation in this text is necessitated by technical attributes of the computer software used to generate the material and adapt it to each individual user.

9. For discussion of the invisibility of female bodies and female experience in medical informatics, see chapter 11.

10. Most systems developed in medical informatics are designed by physicians to support their own work; the field might more accurately be called physician informatics. Not surprisingly, nurses are now developing a parallel field of nursing informatics (ch. 11; Department of Health and Human Services 1993).

11. Compare reference to such a secret fear in Good (1992: 62).

12. A different set of assumptions could have led to a different problem formulation and thus a different migraine system. For example, the team could have envisioned a system that would have—without privileging either perspective—supported the exchange of information between physicians and migraine sufferers by explaining to each some things likely to be taken for granted by the other. Such a system surely would have made more use of our ethnographic finding than the system actually built.

13. The case of the migraine system raises broader issues of agency and intentionality that deserve fuller treatment on their own in relation to this material. Perhaps the most interesting from a science studies standpoint is the extent to which one might want to treat the system itself as an actor (or "actant," to use Latour's term) in relation to its users. To the builders of the migraine system, for whom the notion of machine intelligence is commonplace, the idea of computer programs as intelligent agents is unproblematic. In contrast, among social scientists, at least some of whom view "machine intelligence" as an oxymoron, the attribution of agency to technology is subject to debate (Amsterdamska 1990; Latour 1987).

## 8. Ethics and Politics of Studying Up

1. I thank Susan Kelly for insightful comments on the paper.

2. This abridged French version and its reception by Wylie's informants are discussed in Wylie (1974: viii–x).

3. This term was used by one of my informants in medical informatics to locate anthropological concerns—not irrelevant, but from his standpoint hardly core issues in design either.

4. Numerous people in this field have asked me to recommend a single article that would enable them to do ethnography. Pointing out that field research takes training and expertise tends to produce disbelief and sometimes hostility. The trivial nature of ethnography as viewed from the physician's perspective is demonstrated by

the number of doctors and computer scientists who—having found valuable the results of ethnographic research in medical informatics—set out to do it themselves.

## 9. *Studying Those Who Study Us*

1. I thank my informants, colleagues, and friends in medical informatics for helping my lengthy inquiry in their field. This paper has benefited from my discussion with Bern Shen.

2. Although the Lundsgaarde book was published by a source not necessarily known to informaticians, the book by Anderson, Aydin, and Jay was put out by Springer-Verlag, a major publisher in medical informatics. This book is on display at every American Medical Informatics Association (AMIA) meeting, next to volumes by many "old boys" in the field. To overlook this book is a major act of oversight.

3. Among the publications that inspired Gorman were Osheroff, Forsythe, Buchanan, Bankowitz, Blumenfeld, and Miller (1991) and Forsythe, Buchanan, Osheroff, and Miller (1992).

4. I did not initiate or promote the Rosenal study, but did spend considerable time trying to teach the first author something about ethnography and reviewing in detail several drafts of his paper. At my request, the methods are described as "ethnographically inspired" rather than "ethnography."

## 10. *It's Just a Matter of Common Sense*

1. I am grateful to Bonnie Nardi and to the anonymous reviewers for helpful comments on an earlier draft of this paper. I also thank my informants and colleagues in the world of software design.

2. This section has some repetitions from ch. 9. The repetitions are eliminated, and new material is retained—ed.

3. Some sentences that repeat from ch. 9 are eliminated here—ed.

## 11. *Disappearing Women in the Social World of Computing*

1. I thank the many people in AI and medical informatics who helped me during this long field study. To protect their privacy, they remain anonymous. In the social science community, I thank Deborah Heath, Ruth Linden, and Livia Polanyi for helpful discussions and comments on earlier drafts of this paper. And finally, I thank my parents.

The writing of this paper has been funded by National Library of Medicine grant LM05299-R01 and by a System Development Foundation Fellowship from the Department of Special Collections, Stanford University. The contents of the paper are solely the responsibility of the author and do not represent the official views of the National Library of Medicine or Stanford University.

2. Elsewhere I have described some of the tacit beliefs and expectations characteristic of practitioners in the field (chs. 1–3; Forsythe 1995).

3. For examples of the tacit male perspective in system design in medical informatics, see ch. 7. One example discussed in that paper is the omission of domestic violence from a system-generated list of possible causes of trauma leading to post-traumatic migraine. Since migraine is a condition that affects mainly women, and women are the main victims of domestic violence, I argue that this omission reflects a male perspective on likely sources of trauma in everyday life.

4. Because medical informatics is such an interdisciplinary field, this discussion should ideally consider every field on which it draws. Since three of the laboratories in which I did fieldwork were associated with departments of computer science, and since many of my informants obtained their doctorates in that field, I present statistics on medical informatics and computer science.

5. This description was offered by a senior male informant, himself an "old boy."

6. I could not tell about the three women listed as holding a Ph.D. alone; the discipline was not given.

7. Except for the names of my parents, the personal names used in the main body of this text are pseudonyms.

8. As Davis-Floyd has pointed out, the unpredictable nature of pregnancy and childbirth may also be experienced as problematic in the workplace by professional women who attempt to maintain a "professional/personal split" (1994: 206–8).

9. Diana's notes indicate that the final sections were still under revision—ed.

10. Diana's notes indicate that she might want to discuss identification with the aggressor at this point.—ed.

## *12. George and Sandra's Daughter, Robert's Girl*

1. I am grateful to Susan Kelly, Deborah Heath, Bern Shen, Mary Poovey, and Kath Weston for insightful discussion and helpful comments on earlier drafts of this paper. My debt to the computer scientists, physicians, and support personnel who became my informants is enormous. I thank them sincerely for their help.

2. The other paper is chapter 11—ed.

3. My parents' papers are stored in the Department of Special Collections at my father's university.

4. In fact, there is a great deal of overlap between the concerns of anthropologists and researchers in AI, a perception common to anthropologists but not always shared on the other side of the disciplinary boundary (ch. 6).

5. The next five paragraphs of the manuscript repeat material from the section "Assimilating Women to the World of Men" in chapter 11, and consequently they are not repeated here—ed.

6. For example, one day in the lab I became conscious of a consistent difference between the way anthropologists and computer scientists undertake the task of ex-

planation. Mathematicians and computer scientists seek to order through simplification; they explain things by taking them out of context. In contrast, anthropologists seek order through adding complexity; we try to explain things by putting them into a larger context. How did I know that? It may have been from participant observation in the lab. Then again, I may have picked it up at the dinner table.

# BIBLIOGRAPHY


Abir-Am, P.

1992 "A Historical Ethnography of a Scientific Anniversary in Molecular Biology: The First Protein X-ray Photography (1984, 1934)." *Social Epistemology* 6 (4): 323–54.

American College of Medical Informatics

1994 "Archives, 1984–1992." *Journal of the American Medical Informatics Association* 1 (1): 81–90.

Amsterdamska, O.

1990 "Surely You Are Joking, Monsieur Latour!" *Science, Technology, and Human Values* 15 (4): 495–504.

Anderson, J. G., and C. E. Aydin

1994 "Overview: Theoretical Perspectives and Methodologies for the Evaluation of Health Care Information Systems." In J. G. Anderson, C. E. Aydin, and S. J. Jay (eds.), *Evaluating Health Care Information Systems*. Thousand Oaks, Calif.: Sage. Pp. 5–29.

Anderson, J. G., C. E. Aydin, and S. J. Jay (eds.)

1994 *Evaluating Health Care Information Systems: Methods and Applications*. Thousand Oaks, Calif.: Sage Publications.

Anderson, J. G., and S. J. Jay (eds.)

1987 *Use and Impact of Computers in Clinical Medicine*. New York: Springer-Verlag.

Ardener, S.

1975 "Introduction." In S. Ardener (ed.), *Perceiving Women*. New York: Wiley. Pp. vii–xxiii.

Bader, G. A., and Nyce J. M.

1991 "Theory and Practice in the Development Community: Is There Room for Cultural Analysis?" Presented to American Anthropological Association, Chicago, November.

Barley, S. R.

1986 "Technology as an Occasion for Structuring: Evidence from Observations of CT Scanners and the Social Order of Radiology Departments." *Administrative Science Quarterly* 31 (1): 78–108.

1994 "Technology and the Future of Work." *Administrative Science Quarterly* 39 (1): 183–6.

Barley, S. R., and B. A. Bechky

1994 "In the Backrooms of Science—The Work of Technicians in Science Labs." *Work and Occupations* 21 (1): 85–126.

Bateson, G.

1958 *Naven.* Stanford: Stanford University Press.

Behar, R.

1993 *Translated Woman.* Boston: Beacon Press.

Behar, R., and D. A. Gordon (eds.)

1995 *Women Writing Culture.* Berkeley and Los Angeles: University of California Press.

Benfer, R. A., and L. Furbee

1989 "Knowledge Acquisition in the Peruvian Andes." *AI Expert* 4 (11): 22–9.

Berg, M.

1997 *Rationalizing Medical Work. Decision Support Techniques and Medical Practices.* Cambridge: MIT Press.

Berreman, G. D.

1972 "'Bringing It All Back Home': Malaise in Anthropology." In D. Hymes (ed.), *Reinventing Anthropology.* New York: Pantheon Books. Pp. 83–98.

Blomberg, J., J. Giacomi, A. Mosher, and P. Swenton-Wall

1993 "Ethnographic Field Methods and their Relation to Design." In D. Schuler and A. Namioka (eds.), *Participatory Design: Principles and Practices.* Hillsdale, N.J.: Erlbaum. Pp. 123–56.

Blomberg, J., and A. Henderson

1990 "Reflections on Participatory Design: Lessons from the Trillium Experience." In J. Carrasco Chew and J. Whiteside (eds.), *Empowering People. Proceedings of CHI 1990.* New York: ACM Press. Pp. 353–9.

Bloor, D.

1976 *Knowledge and Social Imagery.* London: Routledge and Kegan Paul.

Boose, J.

1986 *Expertise Transfer for Expert System Design.* New York: Elsevier.

Bourdieu, Pierre

1977 *Outline of a Theory of Practice.* Cambridge: Cambridge University Press.

Buchanan, B.

1988 "Artificial Intelligence as an Experimental Science." In J. H. Fetzer (ed.), *Aspects of Artificial Intelligence.* Norwell, Mass.: Kluwer. Pp. 209–50.

Buchanan, B., D. Barstow, R. Bechtal, J. Bennett, W. Clancey, C. Kulikowski, T. Mitchell, and D. Waterman

1983 "Constructing an Expert System." In F. Hayes-Roth, D. A. Waterman, and D. B. Lenat (eds.), *Building Expert Systems.* Reading, Mass.: Addison-Wesley. Pp. 127–67.

Buchanan, B. G., J. D. Moore, D. E. Forsythe, G. Carenini, S. Ohlsson, and
G. Banks
1995 "An Intelligent Interactive System for Delivering Individualized Information
to Patients." *Artificial Intelligence in Medicine* 7 (2): 117–54.
Buchanan, B., and E. Shortliffe (eds.)
1984 *Rule-Based Expert Systems*. Reading, Mass.: Addison-Wesley.
Callon, M.
1987 "Society in the Making: The Study of Technology as a Tool for Sociological
Analysis." In Wiebe Bijker, Thomas Hughes, and Trevor Pinch (eds.), *The
Social Construction of Technological Systems*. Cambridge: MIT Press.
Pp. 83–103.
Callon, M., J. Law, and A. Rip (eds.)
1986 *Mapping the Dynamics of Science and Technology*. London: Macmillan.
Casper, M. J., and M. Berg
1995 "Introduction to Special Issue on Constructivist Perspectives on Medical
Work: Medical Practices and Science and Technology Studies." *Science,
Technology, and Human Values* 20 (4): 395–407.
Cassell, J., and S. Jacobs (eds.)
1987 *Handbook on Ethical Issues in Anthropology*. Special publication 23 of the
American Anthropological Association. Washington, D.C.: American
Anthropological Association.
Cicourel, A.
1990 "The Integration of Distributed Knowledge in Collaborative Medical Diagno-
sis." In J. Galegher, R. E. Kraut, and C. Egido (eds.), *Intellectual Teamwork.
Social and Intellectual Foundations of Cooperative Work*. Hillsdale, N.J.:
Lawrence Erlbaum. Pp. 221–42.
Clarke, A., and M. Casper
1991 "Making the Wrong Tool for the Job the Right One: Pap Smear Screening
c. 1940–1990." Presented to the Society for Social Studies of Science,
Cambridge, Mass., November.
Clarke, A., and J. Fujimura
1992 *The Right Tools for the Job: At Work in 20th Century Life Sciences*.
Princeton: Princeton University Press.
Coble, J. M., J. S. Maffitt, M. J. Orland, and M. G. Kahn
1995 "Contextual Inquiry: Discovering Physicians' True Needs." In R. M. Gardner
(ed.), *Proceedings of AMIA Annual Fall Symposium*. Philadelphia: Hanley
and Belfus. Pp. 469–73.
Coiera, E.
1996 "Clinical Communication: A New Informatics Paradigm." In J. J. Cimino
(ed.), *Proceedings of AMIA Annual Fall Symposium*. Philadelphia: Hanley
and Belfus. Pp. 17–21.
Cole, J. W.
1977 "Anthropology Comes Part-Way Home: Community Studies in Europe."

In B. J. Siegel, A. R. Beals, and S. A. Tyler (eds.), *Annual Review of Anthropology*. Palo Alto: Annual Reviews. Pp. 349–78.

Collins, H.

1985 *Changing Order: Replication and Induction in Scientific Practice*. Beverly Hills: Sage.

1987a "Expert Systems, Artificial Intelligence and the Behavioural Co-ordinates of Skill." In B. Bloomfield (ed.), *The Question of Artificial Intelligence: Philosophical and Sociological Perspectives*. London: Croom Helm. Pp. 258–82.

1987b "Expert Systems and the Science of Knowledge." In W. Bijker, T. Hughes, and T. Pinch (eds.), *The Social Construction of Technological Systems: New Directions in the Sociology and History of Technology*. Cambridge: MIT Press. Pp. 329–48.

1990 *Artificial Experts: Social Knowledge and Intelligent Machines*. Cambridge: MIT Press.

1992 "AI-VEY!: Response to Slezak." *Social Studies of Science* 22 (1): 201–3.

Collins, H. M., R. H. Green, and R. C. Draper

1985 "Where's the Expertise? Expert Systems as a Medium of Knowledge Transfer." In M. Merry (ed.), *Expert Systems 85*. Cambridge: Cambridge University Press. Pp. 323–34.

Crevier, D.

1993 *AI: The Tumultuous History of the Search for Artificial Intelligence*. New York: Basic Books.

Davis, R.

1989 "Expert Systems: How Far Can They Go?" (2-part article) *AI Magazine* 10 (1): 61–7 and 10 (2): 65–7.

Davis-Floyd, R. E.

1994 "Mind Over Body." In N. Sault (ed.), *Many Mirrors. Body Image and Social Relations*. New Brunswick, N.J.: Rutgers University Press. Pp. 204–33.

Department of Health and Human Services (DHHS)

1993 *Nursing Informatics: Enhancing Patient Care. A Report of the NCNR Priority Expert Panel on Nursing Informatics (National Center for Nursing Research)*. Bethesda, Md.: National Institutes of Health.

Downey, G.

1988 "Structure and Practice in the Cultural Identities of Scientists: Negotiating Nuclear Wastes in New Mexico." *Anthropological Quarterly* 61 (1): 26–38.

Dresselhaus, M. S., J. R. Franz, and B. C. Clark

1994 "Interventions to Increase the Participation of Women in Physics." *Science* 263 (March 11): 1392–3.

Dreyfus, H. L.

1979 *What Computers Can't Do: The Limits of Artificial Intelligence*, rev. ed. New York: Harper and Row.

Dreyfus, H. L., and S. Dreyfus
1986 "Why Computers May Never Think Like People." *Technology Review* 4 (11): 42–61.
Edwards, P. N.
1990 "The Army and the Microworld: Computers and the Politics of Gender Identity." *Signs* 61 (1): 102–27.
Ellen, R.
1984 *Ethnographic Research*. London: Academic Press.
Emerson, R. M., R. I. Fretz, and L. L. Shaw
1995 *Writing Ethnographic Fieldnotes*. Chicago: University of Chicago Press.
Etzkowitz, H., C. Kemelgor, M. Neuschatz, B. Uzzi, and J. Alonzo
1994 "The Paradox of Critical Mass for Women in Science." *Science* 266 (October 7): 51–4.
Fafchamps, D.
1991 "Ethnographic Workflow Analysis: Specifications for Design." In J. H. Bullinger (ed.), *Proceedings of the 4th International Conference on Human-Computer Interaction*. Amsterdam: Elsevier Science Publishers. Pp. 709–15.
Fafchamps, D., C. Y. Young, and P. C. Tang
1991 "Modelling Work Practices: Input to the Design of a Physician Workstation." In P. D. Clayton (ed.), *Proceedings of the 15th Symposium on Computer Applications in Medical Care (SCAMC)*. New York: McGraw-Hill. Pp. 788–92.
Feigenbaum, E.
1985 "Forward." In H. C. Mishkoff (ed.), *Understanding Artificial Intelligence*. Dallas, Tex.: Texas Instruments Information Publishing Center. P. v.
Feigenbaum, E., and P. McCorduck
1984 *The Fifth Generation*. New York: Signet.
Feigenbaum, E., P. McCorduck, and H. P. Nii
1988 *The Rise of the Expert Company: How Visionary Companies Are Using Artificial Intelligence to Achieve Higher Productivity and Profits*. New York: Random House.
Female Graduate Students and Research Staff in the Laboratory for Computer Science and the Artificial Intelligence Laboratory at MIT
1983 *Barriers to Equality in Academia: Women in Computer Science at MIT*. Internal report, Laboratory for Computer Science and Artificial Intelligence Laboratory, Massachusetts Institute of Technology, Cambridge, February.
Fischer, P. J., W. C. Stratmann, H. P. Lundsgaarde, and D. J. Steele
1987 "User Reaction to PROMIS: Issues Related to Acceptability of Medical Innovations." In J. Anderson and S. Jay (eds.), *Use and Impact of Computers in Clinical Medicine*. New York: Springer-Verlag. Pp. 284–301.
Fleck, J.
1994 "Knowing Engineers?: A Response to Forsythe." *Social Studies of Science* 24: 105–13.

Forsythe, D. E.

1989a "Comments on Sherry Turkle's Keynote Address." Presented to the annual conference of the Society for Social Studies of Science, Costa Mesa, California, November 18.

1989b "German Identity and the Problem of History." In E. Tonkin, M. McDonald, and M. Chapman (eds.), *History and Ethnicity*, Association for Social Anthropology Monograph 27. London and New York: Routledge. Pp. 137–56.

1993 "Engineering Knowledge: The Construction of Knowledge in Artificial Intelligence." *Social Studies of Science* 23: 445–77.

1994 "STS (Re)constructs Anthropology: A Reply to Fleck." *Social Studies of Science* 24: 113–23.

1995 "Using Ethnography in the Design of an Explanation System." *Expert Systems With Applications* 8 (4): 403–17.

Forsythe, D. E., and B. G. Buchanan

1989 "Knowledge Acquisition for Expert Systems: Some Pitfalls and Suggestions." *IEEE Transactions on Systems, Man and Cybernetics* 19 (3): 435–42.

1991 "Broadening Our Approach to Evaluating Medical Information Systems." In P. D. Clayton (ed.), *Proceedings of the 15th Symposium on Computer Applications in Medical Care* (SCAMC 91). New York: McGraw-Hill. Pp. 8–12.

1992 "Non-Technical Problems in Knowledge Engineering: Implications for Project Management." *Expert Systems with Applications* 5: 203–12. (Earlier version in J. Liebowitz [ed.], *Proceedings of the World Congress of Expert Systems*. New York: Pergamon, 1991. Pp. 569–77.)

Forsythe, D. E., B. G, Buchanan, J. A. Osheroff, and R. A. Miller

1992 "Expanding the Concept of Medical Information: An Observational Study of Physicians' Information Needs." *Computers and Biomedical Research* 25 (2): 181–200.

Frankel, R. M.

1989 "Talking in Interviews: A Dispreference for Patient-Initiated Questions in Physician-Patient Encounters." In G. Psathas (ed.), *Interaction Competence*. Lanham, Md.: University Press of America. Pp. 231–62.

Fuchs, V. R.

1968 "The Growing Demand for Medical Care." *New England Journal of Medicine* 279: 190–5.

1974 *Who Shall Live? Health, Economics and Social Choice*. New York: Basic Books.

Fujimura, J.

1987 "Constructing 'Do-able' Problems in Cancer Research: Articulating Alignment." *Social Studies of Science* 17: 257–93.

Galegher, J., and R. E. Kraut

1990 "Technology for Intellectual Teamwork: Perspectives on Research and Design." In J. Galegher, R. E. Kraut, and C. Egido (eds.), *Intellectual Teamwork. Social and Technological Foundations of Cooperative Work*. Hillsdale, N.J.: Lawrence Erlbaum. Pp. 1–20.

Garfinkel, H.
1967 *Studies in Ethnomethodology.* Englewood Cliffs, N.J.: Prentice Hall.
Gasser, L.
1986 "The Integration of Computing and Routine Work." *ACM Transactions on Office Information Systems* 4 (3): 205–25.
Geertz, C.
1973 *The Interpretation of Cultures.* New York: Basic Books.
1983 *Local Knowledge.* New York: Basic Books.
1988 *Works and Lives: The Anthropologist as Author.* Stanford: Stanford University Press.
Georgescu-Roegen, N.
1971 *The Entropy Law and the Economic Process.* Cambridge: Harvard University Press.
Goffman, E.
1963 *Stigma: Notes on the Management of Spoiled Identity.* Englewood Cliffs, N.J.: Prentice-Hall.
Good, M.-J.D.
1992 "Work as a Haven From Pain." In M-J. D. Good, P. E. Brodwin, B. J. Good, and A. Kleinman (eds.), *Pain As Human Experience: An Anthropological Perspective.* Berkeley and Los Angeles: University of California Press. Pp. 49–76.
Good, M., P. E. Brodwin, B. J. Good, and A. Kleinman (eds.)
1992 *Pain as Human Experience: An Anthropological Perspective.* Berkeley and Los Angeles: University of California Press.
Gordon, D. R.
1988 "Tenacious Assumptions in Western Medicine." In M. Lock and D. R. Gordon (eds.), *Biomedicine Examined.* Dordrecht: Kluwer. Pp. 19–56.
Gordon, R.
1987 *Interviewing.* Homewood, Ill.: Dorsey Press.
Gorman, P. N., J. Ash, and L. Wykoff
1994 "Can Primary Care Physicians' Questions be Answered Using the Medical Journal Literature?" *Bulletin of the Medical Library Association* 82 (2): 140–6.
Gorman, P. N., and M. Helfand
1995 "Information Seeking in Primary Care: How Physicians Choose Which Clinical Questions to Pursue and Which to Leave Unanswered." *Medical Decision Making* 15 (2): 113–9.
Graves, W., and J. M. Nyce
1992 "Normative Models and Situated Practice in Medicine." *Information and Decision Technologies* 18: 143–9.
Greenbaum, J., and M. Kyng
1991 *Design at Work: Cooperative Design of Computer Systems.* Hillsdale, N.J.: Lawrence Erlbaum.

Gries, D., and D. Marsh
1992 "Taulbee Survey Report: 1989–1990." *Communications of the ACM*
     35 (1): 133–43.
Guha, R. V., and D. B. Lenat
1990 "CYC: A Midterm Report." *A.I. Magazine* 11 (3): 32–59.
Gusterson, H.
1992 "The Rituals of Science: Comments on Abir-Am." *Social Epistemology*
     6 (4): 373–79.
Hakken, David
1999 *Cyborgs@Cyberspace?* New York: Routledge.
Haraway, D.
1989 *Primate Visions.* New York: Routledge.
1991 *Simians, Cyborgs, and Women. The Reinvention of Nature.* New York:
     Routledge.
Harmon, P., and D. King
1985 *Expert Systems.* New York: John Wiley.
Hart, A.
1986 *Knowledge Acquisition for Expert Systems.* New York: McGraw-Hill.
Hayes-Roth, F., D. Waterman, and D. Lenat (eds.)
1983 *Building Expert Systems.* Reading, Mass.: Addison-Wesley.
Hess, D.
1991 *Spirits and Scientists: Ideology, Spiritism, and Brazilian Culture.* University
     Park, Penn.: Pennsylvania State Press.
1992 "Introduction: The New Ethnography and the Anthropology of Science
     and Technology." In D. Hess and L. Layne (eds.), *Knowledge and Society:
     The Anthropology of Science and Technology.* Greenwich, Conn.: JAI Press.
     Pp. 1–26.
1995 *Science and Technology in a Multicultural World.* New York: Columbia
     University Press.
Hess, D., and L. Layne (eds.)
1992 *The Anthropology of Science and Technology.* Greenwich, Conn.: JAI Press.
Hill, R.
1986 "Automating Knowledge Acquisition from Experts." MCC Technical
     Report Number AI-082–86. Austin, Tex.: Microelectronics and Computer
     Technology Corporation.
Hoffman, R. R. (ed.)
1992 *The Psychology of Expertise.* New York: Springer-Verlag.
Hogle, Linda, and Gary Downey (eds.)
1999 "Working for Them: Essays in Honor of Diana Forsythe." *Anthropology of
     Work Review* 20 (1): 1–34.
Howard, R. A., and J. E. Matheson
1984 *Readings on the Principles and Applications of Decision Analysis,* 2nd ed.
     Menlo Park, Calif.: Strategic Decisions Group.

Hunt, L. M., B. Jordan, S. Irwin, and C. H. Browner
1989 "Compliance and the Patient's Perspective: Controlling Symptoms in Everyday Life." *Culture, Medicine and Psychiatry* 13: 315–34.

Johnson, G.
1986 *Machinery of the Mind. Inside the New Science of Artificial Intelligence.* New York: Times Books.

Kahn, R., and D. Cannell
1961 *The Dynamics of Interviewing.* London: Wiley.

Kaplan, B.
1983 "The Computer as Rorschach: Implications for Management and User Acceptance." In R. E. Dayhoff (ed.), *Proceedings of the Seventh Annual Symposium on Computer Applications in Medical Care.* Silver Springs, Md.: IEEE Computer Society.
1987 "The Influence of Medical Values and Practices on Medical Computer Applications." In J. Anderson and S. Jay (eds.), *Use and Impact of Computers in Clinical Medicine.* New York: Springer-Verlag. Pp. 39–50.

Kaplan, B., and D. Duchon
1988 "Combining Qualitative and Quantitative Methods in Information Systems Research: A Case Study." *MIS Quarterly* 12 (4): 571–86.

Kaplan, B., and J. A. Maxwell
1994 "Qualitative Research Methods for Evaluating Computer Information Systems." In J. G. Anderson, C. E. Aydin, and S. J. Jay (eds.), *Evaluating Health Care Information Systems.* Thousand Oaks, Calif.: Sage. Pp. 45–68.

Karp, P. D., and Wilkins, D. C.
1989 "An Analysis of the Distinction Between Deep and Shallow Expert Systems." *International Journal of Expert Systems* 1 (2): 1–32.

Keller, Evelyn Fox
1977 "The Anomaly of a Woman in Physics." In S. Ruddick and P. Daniels (eds.), *Working It Out.* New York: Pantheon Books. Pp. 77–91.
1983 *A Feeling for the Organism: The Life and Work of Barbara McClintock.* New York: W. H. Freeman.

Kidd, A.
1987 "Knowledge Acquisition—An Introductory Framework." In A. Kidd (ed.), *Knowledge Acquisition for Expert Systems. A Practical Handbook.* New York: Plenum Press. Pp. 1–16.

Kirmayer, L. J.
1988 "Mind and Body as Metaphors: Hidden Values in Biomedicine." In M. Lock and D. R. Gordon (eds.), *Biomedicine Examined.* Dordrecht: Kluwer. Pp. 57–93.

Knorr-Cetina, K.
1981 *The Manufacture of Knowledge: An Essay on the Constructivist and Contextual Nature of Science.* New York: Pergamon Press.

Knorr-Cetina, K., and K. Amann
1990 "Image Dissection in Natural Scientific Inquiry." *Science, Technology, and Human Values* 15 (3): 259–83.
Koenig, B. A.
1988 "The Technological Imperative in Medical Practice: The Social Creation of a 'Routine' Treatment." In M. Lock and D. R. Gordon (eds.), *Biomedicine Examined*. Dordrecht: Kluwer. Pp. 465–96.
Kramer, P. E., and S. Lehman
1990 "Mismeasuring Women: A Critique of Research on Computer Ability and Avoidance." *Signs* 16 (1): 158–72.
Kuhn, T.
1970 *The Structure of Scientific Revolutions*, 2nd ed. Chicago: University of Chicago Press.
Lane, P. L., B. A. McLellan, and C. J. Baggoley
1989 "Comparative Efficacy of Chlorpromazine and Meperidine with Dimenhydrinate in Migraine Headache." *Annals of Emergency Medicine* 18: 360–5.
Latour, B.
1987 *Science in Action*. Milton Keynes and Philadelphia: Open University Press.
Latour, B., P. Mauguin, and G. Teil
1992 "A Note on Socio-Technical Graphs." *Social Studies of Science* 22 (1): 33–57.
Latour, B., and S. Woolgar
1986 *Laboratory Life: The Social Construction of Scientific Facts*. Princeton: Princeton University Press.
Law, J.
1987 "Technology and Heterogenous Engineering: The Case of the Portuguese Expansion." In Wiebe Bijker, Thomas Hughes, and Trevor Pinch (eds.), *The Social Construction of Technological Systems*. Cambridge: MIT Press. Pp. 11–34.
Layne, L. (ed.)
1988 "Special Issue: Anthropological Approaches to Science and Technology." *Science, Technology, and Human Values* 23 (1): 3–128.
Lenat, D. G., and E. Feigenbaum
1987 "On the Thresholds of Knowledge." In *Proceedings of the Tenth International Joint Conference on Artificial Intelligence (IJCAI-87)*. Los Altos, Calif.: Morgan Kaufmann. Pp. 1173–82.
Lenat, D. G., and R. V. Guha
1990 *Building Large Knowledge-Based Systems: Representation and Inference in the CYC Project*. Reading, Mass.: Addison-Wesley.
Lenat, D. G., M. Prakash, and M. Shepherd
1986 "CYC: Using Common-Sense Knowledge to Overcome Brittleness and Knowledge Acquisition Bottlenecks." *AI Magazine* 6 (4): 65–85.
Linden, R.
1993 *Making Stories, Making Selves*. Columbus: Ohio State University Press.

Lindenbaum, S., and M. Lock (eds.)

1993 *Knowledge, Power and Practice: The Anthropology of Medicine and Everyday Life.* Berkeley and Los Angeles: University of California Press.

Lock, M., and D. Gordon (eds.)

1988 *Biomedicine Examined.* Dordrecht: Kluwer.

Lundsgaarde, H. P.

1987 "Evaluating Medical Expert Systems." *Social Science and Medicine* 24 (10): 805–19.

Lundsgaarde, H. P., P. J. Fischer, and D. J. Steele

1981 *Human Problems in Computerized Medicine.* Lawrence, Kans.: University of Kansas Publications in Anthropology No. 13.

Lynch, M.

1985 *Art and Artifact in Laboratory Science: A Study of Shop Work and Shop Talk in a Research Laboratory.* Boston: Routledge and Kegan Paul.

McCarthy, J.

1984 "Some Expert Systems Need Common Sense." *Annals of the New York Academy of Sciences* 426: 817–25.

McGrayne, S. B.

1993 *Nobel Prize Women in Science.* New York: Birch Lane Press.

Marcus, G. E., and M. M. J. Fischer

1986 *Anthropology as Cultural Critique.* Chicago: University of Chicago Press.

Miller, J.

1988 "The Role of Human-Computer Interaction in Intelligent Tutoring Systems." In M. Polson and J. Richardson (eds.), *Foundations of Intelligent Tutoring Systems.* Hillsdale, N.J.: Lawrence Erlbaum. Pp. 143–89.

Minnich, E. K.

1990 *Transforming Knowledge.* Philadelphia: Temple University Press.

Minsky, M.

1988 *The Society of Mind.* New York: Simon and Schuster. (First published 1985.)

Morgen, S.

1989 "Gender and Anthropology: Introductory Essay." In S. Morgen (ed.), *Gender and Anthropology.* Washington, D.C.: American Anthropological Association. Pp. 1–20.

Murray, James

1972 *Shorter Oxford English Dictionary.* Oxford: Oxford University Press.

Nader, L.

1972 "Up the Anthropologist—Perspectives Gained From Studying Up." In D. Hymes (ed.), *Reinventing Anthropology.* New York: Random House. Pp. 284–311.

1977 "Studying Up." *Psychology Today* 11 (September): 132.

1980 "The Vertical Slice, Hierarchies and Children." In G. M. Britan and R. Cohen (eds.), *Hierarchy and Society: Anthropological Perspectives on Bureaucracy.* Philadelphia: Institute for the Study of Human Issues. Pp. 31–43.

Nardi, B.
1997 "The Use of Ethnographic Methods in Design and Evaluation." In M. G. Helander, T. Landauer, and P. Prabhu (eds.), *Handbook of Human-Computer Interaction II*. Amsterdam: Elsevier. Pp. 361–6.

Nardi, B., and Y. Engeström
1999 Special Issue: "A Web on the Wind: The Structure of Invisible Work." *Computer Supported Collaborative Work: The Journal of Collaborative Computing* 8: 1–2.

National Science Foundation
1990 *Women and Minorities in Science and Engineering*. Arlington, Va.: National Science Foundation.

Nyce, J., and G. Bader
1993 "Fri att valja? Hierarki, individualism och hypermedia vid tva amerikanska gymnasier" (Hierarchy, Individualism and Hypermedia in Two American High Schools). In L. Ingelstam and L. Sturesson (eds.), *Brus over Landet. Om Informationsoverflodet, kunskapen och Manniskan*. Stockholm: Carlsson. Pp. 247–59.

Nyce, J. M., and W. Graves
1990 "The Construction of Knowledge in Neurology: Implications for Hypermedia System Development." *Artificial Intelligence in Medicine* 2: 315–22.

Nyce, J. M., and J. Lowgren
1995 "Towards Foundational Analysis in Human Computer Interaction." In P. J. Thomas (ed.), *Social and Interactional Dimensions of Human-Computer Interfaces*. Cambridge: Cambridge University Press. Pp. 37–47.

Nyce, J. M, and T. Timpka
1993 "Work, Knowledge, and Argument in Specialist Consultations: Incorporating Tacit Knowledge into System Design and Development." *Medical and Biological Engineering and Computing* 31 (1): HTA 16–9.

Okely, J., and H. Callaway (eds.)
1992 *Anthropology and Autobiography*. ASA Monograph No. 29. London and New York: Routledge.

Olson, J., and H. Rueter
1987 "Extracting Expertise from Experts: Methods for Knowledge Acquisition." *Expert Systems* 4 (3): 152–68.

Osheroff, J. A., D. E. Forsythe, B. G. Buchanan, R. A. Bankowitz, B. H. Blumenfeld, and R. A. Miller
1991 "Physicians' Information Needs: Analysis of Clinical Questions Posed During Clinical Teaching." *Annals of Internal Medicine* 14 (7): 576–81.

Paget, M. A.
1988 *The Unity of Mistakes: A Phenomenological Interpretation of Medical Work*. Philadelphia: Temple University Press.

1993 *A Complex Sorrow: Reflections on Cancer and an Abbreviated Life*. Philadelphia: Temple University Press.

Partridge, D.
1987 "Workshop on the Foundations of AI: Final Report." *AI Magazine* 8 (1): 55–9.
Pearl, A., M. E. Pollack, E. A. Riskin, B. Thomas, E. Wolf, and A. Wu
1990 "Becoming a Computer Scientist: A Report by the ACM Committee on the Status of Women in Computer Science." *Communications of the ACM* 33 (11): 47–57.
Perry, R., and L. Greber
1990 "Women and Computers: An Introduction." *Signs* 16 (1): 74–101.
Pfaffenberger, B.
1988 "Fetishised Objects and Humanised Nature: Towards an Anthropology of Technology." *Man* 23 (2): 236–52.
1992 "The Social Anthropology of Technology." *Annual Review of Anthropology* 21: 491–516.
Polanyi, L.
1995 "Cornucopions of History: A Memoir of Science and the Politics of Private Lives." In G. Marcus (ed.), *Technoscientific Imaginaries: Conversations, Profiles and Memoirs*. Chicago: University of Chicago Press. Pp. 13–43.
Polanyi, M.
1965 *The Tacit Dimension*. New York: Doubleday.
Powdermaker, H.
1966 *Stranger and Friend*. New York: W. W. Norton.
Rapp, Rayna
1993 "Accounting for Amniocentesis." In S. Lindenbaum and M. Lock (eds.), *Knowledge, Power and Practice: The Anthropology of Medicine and Everyday Life*. Berkeley and Los Angeles: University of California Press. Pp. 55–76.
Rosaldo, R.
1993 *Culture and Truth*. Boston: Beacon Press.
Rosenal, T. W., D. E. Forsythe, M. A. Musen, and A. Seiver
1995 "Support for Information Management in Critical Care: A New Approach to Identify Needs." In *AMIA Annual Fall Symposium* (formerly SCAMC). Philadelphia: Hanley and Belfus. Pp. 2–6.
Sachs, P.
1994 "Thinking Through Technology: The Relationship of Technology and Knowledge at Work." Unpublished paper.
Sanjek, R. (ed.)
1990 *Fieldnotes. The Makings of Anthropology*. Ithaca, N.Y.: Cornell University Press.
Saper, J. R., S. D. Silberstein, C. D. Gordon, and R. L. Hamel
1993 *Handbook of Headache Management: A Practical Guide to Diagnosis and Treatment of Head, Neck, and Facial Pain*. Baltimore: Williams and Wilkins.
Scott, A. C., J. E. Clayton, and E. L. Gibson
1991 *A Practical Guide to Knowledge Acquisition*. Reading, Mass.: Addison-Wesley.

Shaw, M., and B. Gaines
1987 "An Interactive Knowledge-Elicitation Technique Using Personal Construct Technology." In A. Kidd (ed.), *Knowledge Acquisition for Expert Systems. A Practical Handbook.* New York: Plenum. Pp. 109–36.

Shields, M. A., W. Graves, and J. M. Nyce
1991 "Technological Innovation in Higher Education: A Case Study in Academic Computing." In J. A. Morell and M. Fleischer (eds.), *Advances in the Implementation and Impact of Computing Systems, Vol. 1.* Greenwich, Conn.: JAI Press. Pp. 183–209.

Shortliffe, E.
1986 "What Is Artificial Intelligence?" *Sumax Report* III.A.2.1. Stanford, Calif.: Knowledge Systems Laboratory, Stanford University.

Shortliffe, E., L. Perreault, G. Wiederhold, and L. Fagan (eds.)
1990 *Medical Informatics: Computer Applications in Health Care.* Reading, Mass.: Addison-Wesley.

Slezak, P.
1989 "Scientific Discovery by Computer as Empirical Refutation of the Strong Program." *Social Studies of Science* 19 (4): 563–600.
1992 "Artificial Experts (Review of Collins)." *Social Studies of Science* 22 (1): 175–201.

Star, S. L.
1989 *Regions of the Mind: Brain Research and the Quest for Scientific Certainty.* Stanford, Calif.: Stanford University Press.
1991 "The Sociology of the Invisible: The Primacy of Work in the Writings of Anselm Strauss." In D. Maines (ed.), *Social Organization and Social Process: Essays in Honor of Anselm Strauss.* New York: Aldine de Gruyter. Pp. 265–83.
1995 "Epilogue: Work and Practice in Social Studies of Science, Medicine, and Technology." *Science, Technology, and Human Values* 20 (4): 501–7.

Stefik, M., and L. Conway
1982 "Toward the Principled Engineering of Knowledge." *AI Magazine* 3 (3): 4–16.

Suchman, L.
1987 *Plans and Situated Actions: The Problem of Human-Machine Communication.* New York: Cambridge University Press.
1990 "Representing Practice in Cognitive Science." In M. Lynch and S. Woolgar (eds.), *Representation in Scientific Practice.* Cambridge: MIT Press. Pp. 301–21.
1992 "Technologies of Accountability: On Lizards and Airplanes." In G. Button (ed.), *Technology in Working Order: Studies of Work, Interaction and Technology.* London: Routledge. Pp. 113–26.
1994 "Located Accountability: Embodying Visions of Technology Production and Use." Presented to the workshop on "Vital Signs: Cultural Perspectives on Coding Life and Vitalizing Code," Stanford University, Calif., June 2–4.

1995 "Making Work Visible." *Communications of the ACM* (9): 56–64.

Tang, P. C., M. A. Jaworski, C. A. Fellencer, N. Kreider, M. P. LaRosa, and W. C. Marquardt

1996 "Clinician Information Activities in Diverse Ambulatory Care Practices." In J. J. Cimino (ed.), *AMIA Annual Fall Symposium* (formerly SCAMC). Philadelphia: Hanley and Belfus. Pp. 12–6.

Tang, P. C., M. A. Jaworski, C. A. Fellencer, M. P. LaRosa, J. M. Lassa, P. Lipsey, and W. C. Marquardt

1995 "Methods for Assessing Information Needs of Clinicians in Ambulatory Care." In R. M. Gardner (ed.), *AMIA Annual Fall Symposium* (formerly SCAMC). Philadelphia: Hanley and Belfus. Pp. 630–4.

Tavris, Carol

1992 *The Mismeasure of Woman*. New York: Simon and Schuster.

Traweek, S.

1988a *Beamtimes and Lifetimes: The World of High Energy Physicists*. Cambridge: Harvard University Press.

1988b "'Feminist Perspectives on Science Studies': Commentary." *Science, Technology, and Human Values* 13(3 and 4): 250–3.

1992 "Border Crossings: Narrative Strategies in Science Studies and among Physicists in Tsukuba Science City, Japan." In A. Pickering (ed.), *Science as Practice and Culture*. Chicago: University of Chicago Press. Pp. 429–65.

Turkle, S.

1988 "Artificial Intelligence and Psychoanalysis: A New Alliance." *Daedalus* 117 (1): 241–68.

1989 "Changing the Subject and Finding the Object: Computation, Gender, and a Sociology of the Concrete." Keynote address presented to the annual conference of the Society for Social Studies of Science, Costa Mesa, California.

Turkle, S., and S. Papert

1990 "Epistemological Pluralism: Styles and Voices within the Computer Culture." *Signs* 16 (1): 128–57.

Visweswaran, K.

1994 *Fictions of Feminist Ethnography*. Minneapolis: University of Minnesota Press.

Wallen, J., H. Waitzkin, and J. D. Stoeckle

1979 "Physician Stereotypes About Female Health and Illness." *Women Health* 4: 371–88.

Waterman, D.

1986 *A Guide to Expert Systems*. Reading, Mass.: Addison-Wesley.

Wax, R. H.

1971 *Doing Fieldwork: Warnings and Advice*. Chicago: University of Chicago Press.

Weinberg, A., L. Ullian, W. Richards, W. and P. Cooper

1981 "Informal Advice- and Information-Seeking Between Physicians." *Journal of Medical Education* 56: 174–80.

Weiss, H. D., B. J. Stern, and J. Goldberg
1991 "Post-traumatic Migraine: Chronic Migraine Precipitated by Minor Head or Neck Trauma." *Headache* 31 (7): 451–6.
Weizenbaum, J.
1976 *Computer Power and Human Reason*. San Francisco: W. H. Freeman.
Werner, O.
1972 "Ethnoscience 1972." In B. Siegel (ed.), *Annual Review of Anthropology*. Palo Alto, Calif.: Annual Reviews. Pp. 271–308.
1978 "The Synthetic Informant Model on the Simulation of Large Lexical/Semantic Fields." In M. Loflin and J. Silverberg (eds.), *Discourse and Inference in Cognitive Anthropology: An Approach to Psychic Unity*. The Hague: Mouton Publishers. Pp. 45–82.
1988 "How to Teach a Network: Minimal Design Features for a Cultural Knowledge Acquisition Device or C-KAD." In M. Evens (ed.), *Relational Models of the Lexicon: Representing Knowledge in Semantic Networks*. Cambridge: Cambridge University Press. Pp. 141–66.
Werner, O., and G. Schoepfle
1987 *Systematic Fieldwork*. Newbury Park, Calif.: Sage.
West, C.
1984 "Medical Misfires: Mishearings, Misgivings, and Misunderstandings in Physician-Patient Dialogues." *Discourse Processes* 7: 107–34.
Whitley, R.
1972 "Black Boxism and the Sociology of Science: A Discussion of the Major Developments in the Field." *Sociological Review Monograph* No. 18, pp. 61–92.
Winograd, T.
1972 *Understanding Natural Language*. Edinburgh: Edinburgh University Press.
Winograd, T., and F. Flores
1986 *Understanding Computers and Cognition: A New Foundation for Design*. Norwood, N.J.: Ablex.
Wolf, E.
1972 "American Anthropologists and American Society." In D. Hymes (ed.), *Reinventing Anthropology*. New York: Pantheon. Pp. 251–63.
Woolgar, S.
1985 "Why Not a Sociology of Machines? The Case of Sociology of Artificial Intelligence." *Sociology* 19: 552–72.
1987 "Reconstructing Man and Machine." In Wiebe Bijker, Thomas Hughes, and Trevor Pinch (eds.), *The Social Construction of Technological Systems*. Cambridge: MIT Press. Pp. 311–28.
1988 *Knowledge and Reflexivity*. London: Sage.
Wylie, L.
1974 *Village in the Vaucluse*, 3rd ed. Cambridge: Harvard University Press.

INDEX

AAAI (American Association for Artificial
Intelligence), 165
Absolute, knowledge seen as, 52
Academic disciplines: cultural dimension of,
16; as intellectual villages, 21
Accountability to informants, 129, 130–31
ACMI (American College of Medical
Informatics), 4, 13, 166, 201
ACORN system, 94, 116
Actants, 62, 206, 209
Action, thought vs., 53
Administration in AI work, 24
Agency, ideas embedded in technology and,
95, 115, 209
AI, *see* Artificial intelligence (AI)
American Anthropological Association, xii,
xix, xx
American Association for Artificial Intelli-
gence (AAAI), 165
American College of Medical Informatics
(ACMI), 4, 13, 166, 201
American Medical Informatics Association
(AMIA), 134, 139, 140, 156, 193, 201,
210
Anderson, J. G., 210
Anthropology: adopting informants'
worldview and, 70, 71–72; appropriation
of, xvii, 69, 207; boundary between
medical informatics and, 143–44; colonial
view of, xvii, 72–74; concerns viewed as
"frosting on the cake," 126, 209; feminist,
119; fieldwork tradition in, 35–36; Fleck's
view of, 69–74; medical, 115; "neutrality"
and, 69–72; positivists' misunderstanding
of, xvii, 136, 140; problem of perspective
in, 69–72, 153–54; working in the U.S.,
119, 120. *See also* Ethnography; Fieldwork; Studying up

*Anthropology of Work Review*, xi–xii, xix
Appropriation of anthropology, xvii, 69, 207
Appropriation of ethnography, xx–xxi,
132–45; bias toward controlled research
and, 135, 137–38; boundary struggles,
143–44; contextual inquiry method, 141;
deletion of ethnographic work, 133,
161–62; dialog reported vs. actual dialog,
154–56; ethnography viewed as common
sense, 135–37, 149, 162; evidence in
AMIA papers, 134, 139, 140–42, 156–57;
fieldwork viewed as talking and reporting,
138, 149, 151; Forsythe's fieldwork
regarding, 132; funding issues, 134,
143–45; informaticians' construction of
ethnography, 134–40; insider status and,
137, 149–50, 154–56; methodology
issues, 137–38, 149, 150–51; misconceptions about ethnography, xxi, 148–52;
patterns viewed as visible and audible,
139–40, 149, 152; positivist vision of
ethnography, 139–42; power issues, xx,
144–45; problems from applying ethnographic misconceptions, 152–57; tacit
knowledge and, 142; verbal presentations
taken for granted, 138–39, 149, 151–52,
195
Ardener, S., 14
Artificial intelligence (AI): Bayesian
approach to, 89–91; boundary disputes
in, 88–92; collective identity of, 75–88;
conscious models taken as real-world
representations in, 10; as context for
study of collective identity and boundary
maintenance, 75–76, 92; culture in
context of, 1–3, 11–12, 202; debate
concerning, 38, 60, 204, 206; definitions
problematic for, 45, 83; engineering ethos

229

# Writing Science